Hearing Impaired Unit

THE DEVELOPMENT OF HEARING

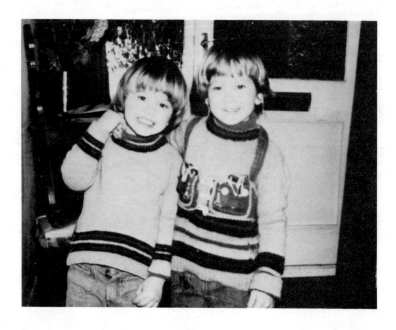

Frontispiece 'The invisible handicap'. The two happy brothers: one has normal hearing but the other is severely deaf

'Frequent returns of deafness incommode me sadly, and half disqualify me for a naturalist; for, when those fits are upon me, I lose all the pleasing notices and little intimations arising from rural sounds: and May is to me . . . silent and mute. . . . And wisdom at one entrance quite shut out.'

Gilbert White, *The Natural History of Selbourne*

Studies in Developmental Paediatrics

Volume 2

THE DEVELOPMENT OF HEARING
Its Progress and Problems

Sybil Yeates

Honorary Consultant Developmental Paediatrician,
Newcomen Centre, Guy's Hospital;
Honorary Consultant in Developmental Paediatrics
(Audiology), Nuffield Centre for Hearing and Speech;
Honorary Consultant, Maudsley and Bethlem Royal
Hospitals

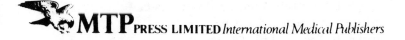
MTP PRESS LIMITED International Medical Publishers

Published by
MTP Press Limited
Falcon House
Lancaster, England

Copyright © 1980 Sybil Yeates

First published 1980

ISBN 0 85200–301–3

Phototypeset in 'Monophoto' Apollo by
Servis Filmsetting Limited, Manchester
Printed in Great Britain by
Butler & Tanner Ltd, Frome

DEDICATION

This book is dedicated to my family for their continuing support and tolerance and love.

It is also dedicated to all the staff of the Hearing and Language Clinic, at The Newcomen Centre, Guy's Hospital, where I think we continue to learn from one another, and to the Director and Staff at the Nuffield Centre for Hearing and Speech, who have inspired and helped me to learn.

CONTENTS

SERIES EDITOR'S NOTE

The discipline of Developmental Paediatrics has highlighted the importance of early life to later performance and adjustment. It is therefore natural that the earliest possible detection of sensory loss, abnormality or malfunction is essential not only for the diagnosis but also for prompt remedial measures.

As in any branch of medicine, diagnosis must precede treatment and the accurate differential diagnosis of hearing loss and language pathology can be one of the most taxing – but rewarding – in developmental paediatrics.

It is fitting that *The Development of Hearing*, the second in the *Studies in Developmental Paediatrics* series, follows volume One – *Language Development and Assessment* – since language and hearing are interwoven.

The overall aim of this series is to provide both a concept of underlying principles and a practical guide to exponents and newcomers alike, and Sybil Yeates, drawing upon her great experience and knowledge, has written a sensitive and commonsense book which more than fulfils this aim.

It deserves to be on the desks of many infant welfare clinics, family doctors' surgeries, and ENT clinics as well as paediatric departments.

Margaret Pollak
Consultant Paediatrician to the Sir Wilfrid Sheldon
Assessment Centre
Senior Lecturer in Developmental, Social and Educational
Paediatrics
King's College Hospital
London SE5

PREFACE

The frontispiece of this book is called 'The invisible handicap'. Most deaf children, with the exception of very unfortunate multiple-handicap children, look quite normal. The young babies who are sent to my clinics for confirmation (or otherwise) of a hearing loss are very often handsome, delightful infants with no other problems.

The deaf child only reveals his handicap when communication is attempted. At that point the picture changes. To an ill-informed observer this child, who had previously seemed quite normal and who had been seen to be playing normally, suddenly appears 'stupid'. That, unhappily, is too often the attitude of the general public towards the deaf person. There is far too often a total misunderstanding of the problems of both the deaf child and the deaf adult.

It must also be admitted that far too often the speech of the deaf is very ugly and when this is added to their difficulties in verbal comprehension we begin to understand why the attitude of the public at large is ill-judged, intolerant and occasionally even hostile.

We must, therefore, aim for three goals. The first must be the ever-increasing education of hearing people about the problems of the deaf, with maximum attempts to involve them with the activities of the deaf community', which has evolved for self-protection and mutual help and understanding, and which must be opened up to sympathetic hearing people.

Secondly we must aim at the early diagnosis and adequate treatment of *every* deaf child. Early diagnosis lies in the hands of the medical profession. Ongoing treatment lies largely with the educationalists, but there is no doubt that children do best where their progress is monitored by a multidisciplinary team. Even when early diagnosis is achieved we cannot be complacent, as this does not necessarily lead to a good 'end product', in other words, a school leaver who can communicate adequately and who can be fully independent and self-supporting in the hearing world, and who can proceed to higher education if he or she is so willed.

This brings me to the third goal. If we are honest we must say that the factors which, together, do produce a good 'end product' are not really well understood. We understand very well many single factors but there are still children who seem to have all the benefits but cannot use them productively, and we do not really understand why this happens, although we find excuses for it. Conversely, there are children who appear to have had few of the benefits but who, nevertheless, make good progress. Hence we need open minds and a big research programme for this small, and I would say 'neglected', section of the community.

In this book I hope to arouse the interest of *all* those people who are concerned with the primary health care of children. If they are actively involved in testing hearing then I hope I can give rise to some 'heartsearching' and consequent improvement of skills. If they are not themselves involved with testing then I hope this book explains the activities of those who do test hearing and shows the enormous importance of such activities. Perhaps even more important would be to remind such colleagues of their vital role in encouraging parents either to accept or, if necessary, seek out really adequate, regular developmental examinations for their children. Many parents mean to do this, and default only through inertia. The all-important query from the family doctor, the health visitor, playgroup leader, the nursery school teacher interviewing before admission, and any of the many doctors who see children in hospital, whether it be casualty officer or consultant, can change inertia into activity, with tremendous effect. In this way *anyone* concerned with paediatric care can help the cause of the child with a hearing loss.

January 1980

Sybil Yeates
Newcomen Centre
Guy's Hospital

ACKNOWLEDGEMENTS

First I must acknowledge a very large debt of gratitude to Mr J.A.M. Martin, Director of the Nuffield Centre for Hearing and Speech, The Royal National Throat, Nose and Ear Hospital. He has been my continuing teacher and friend, and a tremendous source of inspiration.

Next I must thank all those who work in the team at the Hearing and Language Clinic in Guy's Hospital, who have given me very great help in many directions during the last six years. The team has consisted of Mr Ellis Douek, Consultant Otologist, Guy's Hospital, Pamela Snowdon, Senior Teacher of the Deaf, ILEA, Yasmin Saklatvala*, Chief Speech Therapist, Guy's Hospital, a number of Senior ENT Registrars, notably Peter Ashcroft and Michael Stearns, our hospital Physicist, Graham Clarke and his assistant Genevieve Spyer; and we have had the invaluable services of our Chief Audiology Technician, Constantis Onisiphorou. May I add that the work done by any team of this nature is of little value unless the work of the Chief Technician and his staff is of high calibre, given willingly to very small and often very difficult children. I am happy to add that we have had such support.

---

* Present address: King's College Health District.

I am particularly grateful to Peter Ashcroft* for his help on the chapter dealing with the anatomy of the ear.

I must also mention the invaluable services of Roger Penniceard, Senior Educational Psychologist for the Hearing Impaired, ILEA, who also acts as psychologist and adviser to the team, and who sees each of our young patients at an appropriate time as part of their total assessment.

I would like to thank the many parents who have, so willingly, allowed me to use photographs of their children and Tim Everleigh of the Medical Photography Department, Guy's Hospital, who has shown enormous skill and patience in producing most of the photographs. I also thank the staff and pupils at Ladymead School, Taunton, Somerset, for allowing me to use photographs taken by my oldest son, Roger Ashelford. My youngest son, William Ashelford, has also skilfully helped me with his diagrams, aided by my middle son, Lawrence.

Lastly I must thank Cilla Tracy, who has so cheerfully and valiantly typed the script, my secretaries Gillian Pugh and Tracey Clifford, who help me all the time, and my husband, who has been a tower of strength.

Sybil Yeates

---

* Present address: Consultant ENT Surgeon, Royal Hampshire County Hospital.

Chapter 1

INTRODUCTORY MATTERS: WHAT IS OUR AIM?

Medical statistics tell us that 1 in 1000 infants are born with a hearing loss so severe that it needs treatment with auditory training and amplification from the moment of diagnosis. I must add straight away that diagnosis should be made within the first year of life. These children also need special education commencing, broadly speaking, some time before the third birthday. In addition, however, there is also another group of children, again probably about 1 in 1000, who have a hearing loss not as severe as the one originally described, but a loss which will certainly be significant throughout the whole of their lives. Many of these children will need some help with amplification and most will need some extra form of educational 'boost' which is discussed below in Chapter 14.

There is also, however, a third group of children who should not be forgotten. Much research on this group has been very revealing, and I feel that it is proper to include discussion of these children in any book that purports to cover the field of deafness in children. These are the one in five children who, on entering primary school at or around the age of $4-4\frac{1}{2}$ years, are found to have a mild recurrent conductive hearing loss. This loss, although mild in nature, has nevertheless been sufficient to affect their acquisition of speech at the normal time or will affect their ability to learn to read at the expected time. Both problems may occur one after the other.

Although I suppose there is now a general acceptance of the fact that 'early' diagnosis of a hearing loss is desirable, I very much doubt whether there is a uniform effort in all parts of the country to achieve this, and, once achieved, whether the caring professions are to any extent aware of the effect of the trauma of such a diagnosis on a family.

We have already, therefore, found two areas which require constant thought and reappraisal.

It seems fitting to commence with some discussion on efforts that are made to achieve early diagnosis. Discussion with colleagues from many different parts of the United Kingdom seems to indicate that such efforts are often organized by the administrators in community health departments and are carried out by the efforts of individual health visitors. It is probably true to say that nothing can equal the efforts of a good health visitor who knows her area and her families. She will 'stop at nothing' in order to achieve attendance for regular developmental check-ups. But the good health visitor must have a good training, and, although developmental paediatrics now finds some place in the Health Visitors' Course, the amount of time available is often pitifully inadequate. In some cases, the main line of training is simply from one generation of health visitors to the next. In this way, lax habits and unsuitable tests arise, are perpetuated and even worsened. When teaching health visitors modern methods, the cry is often heard 'But they don't do it like that at my clinic'. The new young health visitor, aware of current trends, may be hesitant to correct her senior or the clinic doctor. Thus, the basis of this service must be the thorough training of the new health visitor, with greater emphasis on child development, and with opportunities for practical experience together with regular in-service refresher courses. Only in this way can we achieve some uniformity of standards throughout the country.

In the same way, it is very necessary to improve the training in developmental paediatrics offered to medical students and doctors. Many young doctors take up paediatric posts without any training in this branch of the speciality. Many doctors are asked 'to do a clinic' without having any idea of the developmental techniques that should be used.

Medical students taking paediatrics should also be taught about the examination of 'well' children in addition to the curing of the sick child. The latter has more glamour and more appeal to the student, but, once qualified, he is more likely to be confronted by the problems of the basically well child, and his training should not leave him incompetent in this respect. In the same way, child health clinics should only be staffed by doctors whose training in this sphere has been adequate.[1] At least there is now a host of postgraduate courses offering this training, and there is a great responsibility on all those who will ever need to test the hearing of infants and young children to offer themselves for re-education in this field.

If, then, we depend basically on the activites of our health visitors, what do we expect of them? What is our aim? Our aim, surely, must be to test the hearing of *every* infant and young child at regular and crucial intervals (see chapter 5), with suitable techniques.

As an aim, nothing could appear more simple – in print or on our lips. In practice, however, this proves *not* the case. I have had the opportunity of comparing the percentages of children examined in different parts of London in 1978. In the first year of life, in an outer London district, 90% of children were estimated to have had their first hearing test at some time between the ages of 7 months and 1 year. In an inner London district, however, only 61% of children were given that first test before their first birthday. What is more, in the latter district, only approximately 47% of children were given the crucial 3-year-old examination (see Chapter 5), and this included the children who were already in nursery school and therefore provided an easy target.

Why is this the case? There are many factors which crop up time and again and which may be briefly considered here. First and foremost is the incredible fact that many mothers are still unaware of the facilities available. Some have heard about 'check-ups' or 'hearing tests' but do not know where to seek them. Others still remain ignorant of the *full* services offered. If my professional colleagues are now expressing disbelief, I commend to them the exercise of talking to any non-professional group and eliciting their comments on this subject.

So the first task remains the offering of such examinations to all families at the relevant times, together with explanations of where and why they are offered. We do not even use our present facilities to their fullest extent. In every district, family doctors, child health doctors, hospital doctors, health visitors and administrators should put together suitable schemes to ensure that the maximum number of children are seen. It should be commonplace for family doctors and paediatricians to enquire about the results of such examinations, to communicate the results to all parties concerned and, when necessary, to commend them to any mother who seems reluctant or apathetic.

We certainly do not make full use of health education departments in this sphere. In my experience, this is a field where they usually express considerable interest in developmental work and often produce posters, leaflets, films, etc. There is no doubt that this is one of the most suitable targets for health education, but, as always, it is only knowledge coupled with enthusiasm that can exploit our facilities. Incidentally, the machinery for this exists and the amount of extra financial outlay required is not great.

What then of the families who know of the opportunities

and fail to use them? In the end, of course, this amounts to a failure to understand the significance of the tests. In many cases, it may be seen as yet another chore that 'they', that is, authority, are forcing upon the busy mother. Hence the multitude of excuses that one hears time after time. 'I know my baby can hear. There's no need to bring him to the clinic/surgery.' When enquiring *how* the family knows the baby can hear, we are told that he looks up when he hears aeroplanes or looks round when he hears traffic. But, in both cases, the sounds referred to have a large low-tone component. Many severely deaf babies have a small island of hearing left in the lower frequencies so these children may hear *some* aeroplane or traffic noises, but, nevertheless, they hear *very little speech*.

Many mothers mean well but never get round to the point of arrival for tests. Perhaps they have other small children, live in a tower block with all the well-known lift problems, or in a rural area with a poor bus service.

In all these cases, we are almost totally reliant upon the quality of the health visitor, her ability to explain and educate, and, in general, her ability to 'move mountains' so that all the children under her care benefit from the available services. In some cases, it may be essential for the developmental/hearing team to visit the patient at home. There are, of course, hazards here in the form of much extraneous noise, other children who wish to 'help' the examiners and so on. However, the presence of difficulties should, hopefully, stimulate the expertise of the health visitor so that she is able to overcome, at least to some extent, each problem as it arises.

In my view, the best time to commence this type of education is when young people are still at school. Both boys and girls should be taught the routines of regular developmental checks with suitable explanations of the need for them. In my experience, the interest of both boys and girls between the ages of 12 and 18 years is considerable. Here again, health education departments are available to help but vary greatly in their usefulness. Certainly there are some departments that produce suitable material and that are very pleased to be asked to participate. I am quite sure that such departments are under-used by family doctors and paediatric departments.

References

1, Joint Paediatric Committee of the Royal Colleges of Physicians and the British Paediatric Association. (1978). *Clinical Medical Officers in the Child Health Service.* (British Paediatric Association) [This offers new ideas on training and career structure for Clinical Medical Officers]

Chapter 2

INFANTS AT RISK

Although we aim at testing *every* baby, we must immediately qualify this by saying that 'all babies are important
but some are more important than others'. Opinions vary
somewhat about which babies should be sought out with the
greatest fervour. All agree, however, that a family history of
deafness is very important. The genes concerned in such a
family history may be autosomal dominant, autosomal
recessive or X-linked (see Chapter 11). In each case, the child
may be completely normal apart from the hearing loss, or, to
use Fraser's term[1], the hearing loss is 'clinically undifferentiated'. On the other hand, the hearing loss may form part of
a recognizable picture, inherited in a recognizable manner,
in which hearing loss is only one part of the general pattern.
In other words, 'syndromes' including hearing loss may be
inherited in all three ways.

The three common* syndromes inherited in autosomal
recessive manner are Pendred's syndrome, Usher's syndrome and the abnormal ECG syndrome or Jervell–Lange–
Neilsen syndrome. The 'common' syndromes inherited in
autosomal dominant manner are the auditory–pigmentary
syndromes. While Fraser[2] found, in a school study in the

---

* The term 'common' is used here in a *very* relative manner
(see Chapters 11 and 12).

British Isles, that 25.2% of severely deaf children came into the category of clinically undifferentiated autosomal recessive inheritance, he found that only 5.7% of children had Pendred's syndrome, 1.2% had Usher's syndrome and 0.7% had abnormal ECG syndrome; 11.6% had clinically undifferentiated autosomal dominant inheritance, while only 3.2% had auditory–pigmentary syndromes. These figures are quoted to underline the necessity of testing all babies where there is even a *remote* family history of hearing loss.

The next very important category is that in which there is a history of infectious illness during pregnancy. The most important culprit is *rubella* (german measles) which may result in not only damage to the cochlea, but extensive damage to the eye (producing cataracts and choroidoretinitis), microcephaly and mental defect, hepatosplenomegaly, thrombocytopenia, etc. The earlier in pregnancy the infection occurs, the greater seems to be the damage. In the survey made by Fraser, to which we have previously referred, he found that 6.4% of cases of severe hearing loss in the school children studied in 1960–61, were due to rubella (Figure 1). But although we now have an effective vaccine against rubella, it is with a feeling of great shame that I have to record another outbreak of rubella in 1978 which will undoubtedly result in another 'generation' of severely handicapped children*. It is to be hoped that family doctors, paediatricians and health visitors will now conduct a major and vigorous campaign to protect all girls and young women. There is little doubt that most women are completely unaware of the appalling possibilities of fetal rubella. I can clearly remember the impact of a severe case of rubella syndrome on a speech therapy student who was attending my clinic. When one considers that she came from a section

---

* A leading article in *The Guardian* (9 April 79), 'Why no action against rubella', made pungent and accurate comments about inertia on this subject.

of society that is considered to be informed in these matters, we then realize the degree of ignorance amongst the public at large. This, again, is where we should enlist the help of the local health education department.

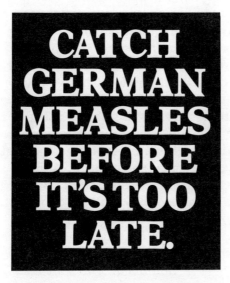

Figure 1   The propaganda that came too late?

Other infectious illnesses in pregnancy, such as mumps and cytomegalovirus (CMV), can also be hazardous. The latter is specially 'deadly' as the mother's illness is minimal, 'a day off colour' perhaps, while the damage to the fetus is enormous. Mental retardation with microcephaly is common, often with damage to the developing eyes. Occasionally the cochlea is also damaged.

Drugs given in pregnancy can be damaging, especially streptomycin and, even more, dihydrostreptomycin and allied drugs. The now commonly adopted rule of avoiding all but essential drugs during pregnancy has cut down this risk.

Premature or 'small for dates' babies are particularly

prone to damage in the cochlea and should be carefully supervised for hearing loss.

Any condition which produces anoxia, around the time of birth, either before, during or just after birth, can also damage the very small and delicate cochlea. The number of conditions producing anoxia are manifold and need not be listed here. Of course, if there is anoxia in a premature baby, the risk becomes even higher.

After birth, the commonest hazard is a raised serum bilirubin in the newborn period. This is usually the result of Rh incompatibility, but may also be the result of AB–O incompatibility or even excessive physiological jaundice in a premature baby. Paediatricians, of course, monitor the serum bilirubin levels very carefully after birth but there is not yet entire agreement about the level which is damaging to the cochlear nuclei. However, work done by Fenwick in Birmingham[3] seemed to show quite conclusively that levels above 15 mg/100 ml *could* be dangerous. This is, of course, a lower figure than that used by many neonatal paediatricians to indicate the necessity for exchange transfusion.

Diseases in early childhood, which are common and can be damaging, include meningitis, measles and mumps. In the latter two cases, fortunately, the effect is generally unilateral, although we should not underrate the inconvenience of severe unilateral hearing loss both to the child and the adult. The child in a class where the teacher walks round as she talks may find himself missing at least some portion of what is going on, and is consequently labelled as 'inattentive', 'dreamy' or 'naughty'. The adult trying to make conversation in a room full of people, or holding a telephone to his 'good' ear while taking instructions from the 'bad' side, can become very stressed.

Around 5% of all cases of meningitis may be left with hearing loss as a sequel. The organism involved or the degree of severity of the illness does not seem to matter. The deafness complicating meningitis is usually very severe indeed. Some of my patients with the most severe degree of hearing handicap are post-meningitics.

If the post-meningitic deaf child is older and has developed speech, the function of the teacher and speech therapist is vital in maintaining as much of the child's language as possible. Although most parents are happy that their child has not succumbed to the illness itself, there are also many families where the disaster of hearing a child's speech deteriorating has enormous emotional repercussions within the family circle. It is necessary to make these parents aware that help is at hand and to involve them actively in the help that is given.

To sum up, then, we may say that our aim is to test the hearing of every baby but we must search out with particular care the categories with the following indications:

(1) Family history of hearing loss.
(2) Any infectious illness in pregnancy.
(3) Use of drugs in pregnancy.
(4) Anoxia, from any cause, around the time of birth.
(5) Premature or small-for-dates babies.
(6) Raised serum bilirubin level in newborn period.
(7) History of meningitis.
(8) Following common infectious illnesses, such as measles or mumps.
(9) Recurrent upper respiratory tract infections, leading to chronic secretory otitis media (see Chapter 15).

All these conditions are dealt with more fully in Chapters 11 and 12. But there is also an important tenth 'rule' to remember. Any child who is not developing speech at the expected rate should have his hearing checked with special care. In fact, it is wise that any such child, showing normal intelligence, should be assumed to be deaf until proved otherwise.

References

1. Fraser, G.R. (1976). *Causes of Profound Deafness in Childhood*, p. 147. (London: Baillière Tindall)
2. Fraser, (1976), pp. 318–319
3. Fenwick, J.D. (1975). Neonatal jaundice as a cause of deafness. *Laryngol. Otol.*, **89**, 925

Chapter 3

THE NATURE OF SOUND

Whenever one begins to talk about hearing, it is necessary to talk about sound. We wish, basically, to know three things about any sound:
  (1) Its frequency or pitch.
  (2) Its volume or intensity.
  (3) Its duration.
We will consider these in turn.

FREQUENCY

The frequency of a sound is simply the number of vibrations or waves, or compressions and rarefactions, that occur in a given medium in a given time. It is usually convenient to talk about the number of complete waves that a sound makes in air in a second. Such a measurement, formerly known as cycles per second (cps), is now known as *hertz* (Hz); that is, one cps = one Hz, 1000 Hz are called a kilohertz (1 kHz) etc.

  The sounds that we hear around us, whether beautiful or ugly, usually contain some interest. This is because they consist of a fundamental or prominent tone which is usually surrounded by numerous overtones stretching across many frequencies. We can, of course, produce pure tones, which we use constantly when testing hearing, but most people will agree that pure tones are very dull when compared with everyday sounds. This is probably the reason why young babies, when tested between 7 months and 1 year, do not turn to pure tones until a much greater volume is produced than that required to obtain the same response with the cup and spoon, rattle and voice (see Chapter 8). This means that, in practice, we do not use a free field audiometer when testing children under 1 year or so.

The frequencies used in speech also cover an enormously wide range. Sheridan[1] estimates this as being between 64 and 8192 Hz. Because the range is so wide, it is convenient to divide it into three sections; up to 500 Hz are known as the low frequencies, from 500 Hz to 2 kHz are the middle frequencies, and above 2 kHz are the high frequencies (Figure 2).

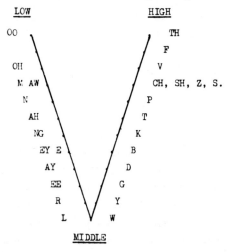

Figure 2   Diagram giving an approximation of the sequence of speech frequencies from low to high frequencies

The low and lower-middle frequencies are important for the purpose of energy in speech and therefore the carrying power and the emotional quality. These tend to be the louder sounds in speech and are found in the vowels.

Thus we can attribute the above qualities to the vowels in our speech. I suggest the reader says two sounds aloud, first a vowel sound such as *aw* and then a consonant sound such as *th*. I think he can then easily appreciate the difference in volume between the vowel and the consonant.

The high-frequency sounds, on the other hand, are immensely important as they are *responsible for the intelligibility of speech*. Another small exercise suggested to the reader is that he takes any small sentence, such as 'The boy lost his dog', and says it aloud, omitting the consonants. He will find it becomes unintelligible. If, on the other hand, he retains the consonants and uses just one neutral vowel sound, such as *er* throughout the sentence, he will find that

Table 1   Diagram of frequencies of speech sounds

Sound	Frequency	Approximate volume in speech
OO	250 Hz	40 dB
AW	375 Hz	45 dB
M	375 Hz	35 dB
N	500 Hz	40 dB
AH	600 Hz (approx.)	50 dB
NG	750 Hz	40 dB
AY	1 kHz	50 + dB
EE	1750 Hz (approx.)	50 dB
D	2 kHz +	35 dB
T	3 kHz (approx.)	35 dB
S	4 kHz	40 dB
F	5 kHz	30–35 dB
TH	6 kHz +	30 dB

although it sounds odd it remains largely intelligible. This gives the reader some idea of what is happening to the child with a high-frequency loss, and also compares his plight with that of the child whose loss is mainly in the lower frequencies and for whom the acquisition of speech is relatively much easier.

The child with a very severe high-frequency loss will neither learn to comprehend speech nor to acquire expressive speech, unless he is given active and very specialized help. The child with a less severe high-frequency loss will probably acquire some expressive language but it will be largely unintelligible to others, although meaningful for himself. He, too, will have tremendous problems in verbal comprehension. Lastly, the child with a very mild high-frequency loss will be in severe difficulties but of a rather different type. He will probably acquire a lot of expressive speech, showing articulation problems associated with his lack of hearing of those consonants in the highest frequency ranges, such as *s, sh, ch, th, f* and *v*. A competent speech therapist, especially if working in conjunction with a teacher of the deaf, can give a lot of very adequate help here. However, the child's difficulties in verbal comprehension form a far more complex problem. This is because, in a child who has acquired a relatively good vocabulary, the brain attempts to compensate for the deficiency of his ears, and thus, attempts to substitute similar high-frequency sounds for the ones that he has heard incorrectly; for example, he may 'hear' the word *dish* instead of *fish, money* instead of *honey*, or *feet* instead of *seat* – the reader can himself think up scores of other examples very quickly.

Added to this is the problem that because the child can hear low frequencies very efficiently he does not appear to be deaf. He turns to a voice even if he has not heard the words accurately, to footsteps behind him, doors shutting, etc. Because of this, parents, and especially teachers, deny vigorously that he is deaf. Instead of this, especially at school, he gets other labels attached to him, such as 'inattentive', 'dreamy', 'disobedient', and 'naughty' in general.

I have had patients labelled as maladjusted and educationally subnormal. In the former case, the little girl of between 4 and 5 years old was intensely withdrawn. There were also problems at home. In the middle of our investigations, she was independently referred to a psychiatrist who informed me that further hearing tests were not necessary as her troubles did not stem from that region. In fact, we completed our tests to find that she had a very marked bilateral high-frequency hearing loss. This was a very handicapped child with both emotional and hearing problems. The latter undoubtedly exacerbated the former and she was finally placed in a unit for the partially hearing with continuing help from the psychiatrist. As for the child who was placed in a school for educationally subnormal pupils, he, too, has proved to have a high-frequency hearing loss together with a *non-verbal* IQ which lies within the superior range. His attainments have, of course, improved markedly since his high-frequency loss, discovered at the age of 9 years, has been treated, with the cooperation of a doctor and teacher of the deaf.

From the above anecdotes, we can draw two important conclusions. First, when a child is brought to your attention because he is 'inattentive', 'withdrawn', 'dreamy', 'lazy' or 'naughty', particularly when he is in a younger age group, it is always wise to test his hearing, even if this is reported as being quite normal. Secondly, when a child has a hearing loss, it is pointless to measure his IQ using verbally based tests. It is not at all uncommon to see children with a hearing loss whose IQ label is based on a Stanford–Binet test, which is very much biased towards verbal tests. Such children's abilities can only be judged by the use of non-verbal tests, such as the Snijders-Oomen test or the non-verbal part of the Wechsler Intelligence Scale for Children (WISC).

VOLUME OR INTENSITY

Whereas the frequency of a sound is measured by the number of waves in a given time, its volume is measured by the amplitude of these waves, and the unit of measurement is known as the *bel*, so called after the inventor of the telephone, Sir Alexander Graham Bell. A bel is, in fact, a very large amount of sound pressure and we therefore normally divide it by 10 and talk about *decibels*. The difference between very soft and very loud sounds is considerable and it may interest the reader to know that a barely decipherable whisper is about a thousand times louder than the very softest sound that can be heard. On the other hand, an ordinary conversational voice is about a million times louder than the same soft sound that is only just audible[2].

The softest sound just deciphered by the human ear is designated 0 dB. For the calibration of audiometers which measure the volume of pure tones, generally between 125 Hz and 8 kHz, a very large sample of the population was taken. The level at which each subject could just detect sounds at each frequency was found, and averages were taken, thus providing a baseline from 125 Hz to 8 kHz.

The important thing to remember about volume of sound in speech is how very loudly most of us talk. A normal conversational voice varies between 30 and 60 dB, the softest sounds being the consonants, particularly the very high-frequency consonants such as *v, f* and *th*, while the loudest sounds are the vowels; the vowels of lowest frequency are *oo, oh* and *aw*. When using speech for hearing tests it is particularly important to remember the volume of our normal conversational voice.

DURATION

This is a small point of interest and some significance.

Common sense indicates that a sound of long duration is easier to hear than a shortlived sound. In a similar way, some of our consonants are of longer duration than others. The reader can compare for himself sounds such as *sh* and *s*, with *t* and *p*, for instance. The former are known as *continuants* and last longer than the latter which are known as short *plosives*. The very nature of the term 'plosive' indicates something short and sharp. However, from Figure 2 the reader can see that *sh* and *s* are of higher frequency than *t* and *p*. Therefore, if we follow the statements already made, we should expect *sh* and *s* to be softer in quality than *t* and *p*. But, because of the increased duration of the continuant consonants, these are, in fact, louder than the short, sharp plosive consonants, which are of rather lower frequency.

References

1. Sheridan, M.D. (1976). *Manual for the Stycar Hearing Tests*. 2nd Edn. (Windsor: NFER Publishing Company)
2. Bloom, F. (1978). *Our Deaf Children into the 80s* (Old Woking: Unwin Brothers, The Gresham Press)

Chapter 4

A PHYSICIAN'S REVISION OF THE ANATOMY OF THE EAR

It is certainly not the intention of this chapter to revise the anatomy of the ear in any great detail. However, when one is actively engaged in testing hearing in young children, the anatomy of this area takes on a new interest.

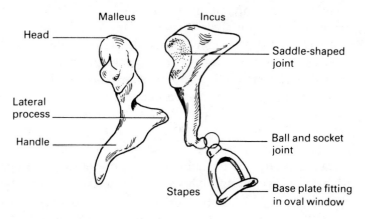

Figure 3   Diagram of the ossicles to show their joints

The external ear in man has a shape that is useful for collecting sound, although this feature is not as marked as it is in many animals, such as the long-eared bat. Neither do we retain the ability to move our external ears to any great extent, except maybe as a party piece! We do, however, retain vestigial postauricular muscles which originally fulfilled this purpose and are of considerable interest. Electrodes placed on almost any muscle in the body show an electrical response to sound stimuli, and this is particularly so in the postauricular muscles where the responses are exceptionally well marked. The responses are still, however, very small and, in order to record them with reasonable accuracy, they must first be summated in an averaging computer. This is the basis of one of the electrical tests of hearing in current use (see Chapter 17).

The canal leading from the external ear to the tympanic membrane is called the *external auditory meatus* and is about 25 mm long in an adult and correspondingly shorter in children. The cuticular lining of the canal is interesting as it contains fine hairs and two sets of glands, the sebaceous glands and ceruminous or wax-producing glands. When examining the tympanic membranes of young infants, the hairs are often relatively long, preventing a really good view of the drum. If they become blocked, the sebaceous glands can become infected and lead to painful 'boils' in the external auditory canal. The wax-producing glands are important as some wax in the canals prevents the lining becoming soggy when water goes into the canals while washing, swimming, etc. Many people become unduly worried about the presence of wax in the ears of children; in general, it should be left alone as it is preferable to an ear with a dry, flaky lining that is so prone to otitis externa. But if it is obviously forming a hard solid plug, which prevents the optimal passage of sound to the tympanic membrane, then it should be removed. Another reason for removal is discomfort, when the child complains that the wax-filled ear 'does not feel like the other ear'.

The best reason for removal, however, is in the deaf child wearing a hearing aid. Wax in the ears of these children often prevents the mould or earpiece attached to the hearing aid fitting snugly in the ear. This in turn leads to the most unacceptable whistling or feedback which is so often associated with the deaf person. This whistling is not caused by a fault in the aid itself, but is due to an ill-fitting mould, and one of the commonest causes of this is the presence of a large plug of wax in the ear. The wax should generally be removed by syringing and a skilled operator is required so that the child is not frightened or hurt. Drops, such as olive oil on a warmed teaspoon, sodium bicarbonate, or a proprietary preparation, should be used for a few days before syringing if the wax is hard. ENT surgeons may, of course, remove the wax under direct vision.

It is interesting and important to remember that the nerve supply of the external auditory meatus includes both the auriculo-temporal branch of the 5th nerve and the auricular branch of the vagus. The latter can be unpleasantly stimulated by a doctor examining an ear with a probe. In fact two hazards can occur. Water that is too cold for syringing can produce an unpleasant and frightening attack when the patient complains of intense giddiness due to the caloric effect. Recovery is rapid when the syringing is immediately ceased. On the other hand, when the surgeon is using a probe, the vagus may be stimulated causing the patient to have a vasovagal attack, in which typically he becomes pale, cold, clammy, nauseated and may faint. Fortunately, neither occurrence is frequent.

The external auditory meatus may be congenitally absent, as may the external ear itself. Sometimes an absent external auditory meatus is associated with accessory auricles which are usually small tags of skin found in front of or just below the normal position of the pinna, such as in Treacher–Collins syndrome or mandibulo-facial dysostosis, oculo-auriculo-vertebral dysplasia, and Moebius syndrome. (These are all rare syndromes but the author has had cases of all three conditions attending her clinic.) In other cases, however, the lesion seems to be isolated and the child is normal in all other respects. The specialist surgeon may be willing to undertake surgical intervention, both to fashion a pinna and also, if bilateral, to open up the external auditory canal. In the latter case, any operation is always preceded by tomograms to see whether the middle and inner ears look reasonably normal. If they are also grossly malformed, there is little point in subjecting a child to surgery when the hearing can not improve further as a result of interference.

At the end of the external auditory canal lies the *tympanic membrane* or *eardrum*. This is a most interesting structure, being both thin and tough in order to fulfil its function adequately. It consists of three layers. The outer layer is cuticular in nature, while the innermost layer is of mucous membrane continuous with that lining the remainder of the middle ear. Between these two layers is a fibrous layer which consists of radial and circumferential fibres. The former run from the centre of the drum or *umbo* to the periphery, and it is this middle layer which gives strength to the tympanic membrane.

It can be seen from this description that, whilst the tympanic membrane is sufficiently delicate to respond to the incoming sound waves by movement, it is also sufficiently tough to withstand changes of pressure within the middle ear. Changes of pressure in the middle ear may result from failure of the eustachian or pharyngo-tympanic tube to open, or during changes in air pressure, such as when in a descending aircraft which often produces temporary feelings of discomfort in the ears. Again, failure of eustachian tube function contributes largely to the formation of sterile serous effusions in the middle ear, which are preceded by a state of negative pressure in the middle ear, in secretory otitis media. On the other hand, infection in the middle ear, with the production of purulent discharge, can also change the pressure in the middle ear, especially if the eustachian tube is blocked by the infective process. In these cases, earache results and treatment is normally

quickly commenced. Before the days of antibiotics, however, rising pressure due to increasing amounts of pus in the
middle ear often ruptured the drum with release of purulent
discharge and relief of the intense earache. Even in those
days the competent doctor attempted to diagnose the
condition before this stage was reached so that a myringotomy, or small slit in the drum, could be made by the
surgeon to release the pressure and discharge before the
drum ruptured spontaneously. A surgical slit heals very
much better than a ragged tear made by the bursting drum.
The latter often resulted in an ear with a chronic troublesome discharge which, fortunately, we rarely see now. This
subject is discussed at greater length in Chapter 15.

The *middle ear* itself, of which the tympanic membrane
forms the lateral boundary, is a very small cavity in the
petrous temporal bone, narrow and slit-like in shape. The
most important thing to remember about the middle ear is
that, in its healthy state, it is an *air-filled* cavity; the pressure
in the healthy middle ear is *air* pressure. This is because on
the anterior wall of the middle ear is the opening of the
eustachian or *pharyngo-tympanic tube*. This, as its name
implies, connects the middle ear with the pharynx, and
normally air passes from the pharynx through the eustachian tube to the middle ear. Unfortunately, as is immediately
obvious, organisms can also pass along this route which is
only about 40 mm long in an adult and relatively shorter in
young children. Again, this is discussed on pp. 185–193.

Above the opening of the eustachian tube, on the anterior
wall of the middle ear, is a canal in which runs the *tensor
tympani* muscle, one of the two small muscles of the middle
ear.

The medial wall of the middle ear separates it from the
inner ear and several important landmarks are found on it.
Firstly, there is a projection which is rounded in nature and
called the *promontory*. This is produced by the first turn of
the cochlea, the shell-like structure of the inner ear. (The

cochlea, as we shall note, contains a central column, surrounded by two-and-a-half spiral turns.) When an electrode is put into the middle ear, as in an electrical hearing test, it is placed on this promontory and can pick up electrical changes in the cochlea. This test is known as an *electrocochleogram* and is briefly mentioned in Chapter 17.

Above the posterior part of the promontory is the oval window or *fenestra vestibuli*. This window is extremely important as it is filled by the base plate of the stapes, the third of the small bones found in the middle ear. It is also covered by mucous membrane but provides a connecting point between the middle and inner ears.

Below the posterior end of the promontory is the round window or *fenestra cochleae* which is covered by the secondary tympanic membrane. This is another point of connection between the middle and inner ears.

There is another rounded ridge on the medial wall of the middle ear, above the promontory and oval window. This is produced by the facial or 7th nerve lying in its bony canal, and surgeons working in the vicinity of the middle and inner ears are always aware of the close proximity of the 7th nerve.

We have now described the lateral, anterior and medial walls of the middle ear. The remaining wall (the posterior wall) connects with the *mastoid antrum* which is a small air-sinus in the posterior bone. It is very important because air cells open out of the antrum. They are connected with one another and burrow into the mastoid process. Thus it can be seen how untreated middle ear conditions can lead to infection in these air cells causing mastoiditis. Also the posterior wall of the antrum separates it from the sigmoid sinus and the cerebellar hemisphere. These facts are only included to remind the reader that the middle ear is closely related to important structures. With the advent of anti-biotics, the dangers of such complications as mastoiditis, thrombosis of the sigmoid sinus and meningitis have largely

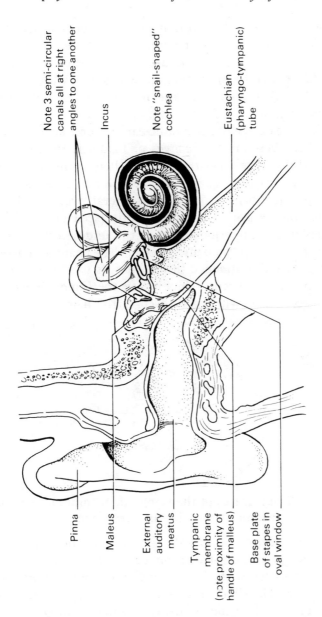

Note 3 semi-circular canals all at right angles to one another

Incus

Note "snail-shaped" cochlea

Eustachian (pharyngo-tympanic) tube

Pinna

Maleus

External auditory meatus

Tympanic membrane (note proximity of handle of malleus)

Base plate of stapes in oval window

Figure 4   The general structure of the ear

disappeared. It is still important to remember that diseases of the middle ear are of very great importance.

The other interesting structure on the posterior wall of the middle ear is the projection known as the *pyramid* from which the other muscle of the middle ear emerges, the *stapedius* muscle.

Within the cavity of the middle ear are three small bones or *ossicles*. These are the *malleus* or hammer, the *incus* or anvil, and the *stapes* or stirrup. The malleus is the largest of the three and consists of a rounded head, a very short neck, a handle or manubrium and a little lateral process which projects from the upper end of the handle (see Figure 3). The head lies in the uppermost part of the middle ear cavity, known as the epitympanic recess. The handle passes downwards and is attached throughout its whole length to the tympanic membrane. Thus, when the tympanic membrane is examined with an auroscope, the hammer handle and lateral process should be clearly seen (Figure 5).

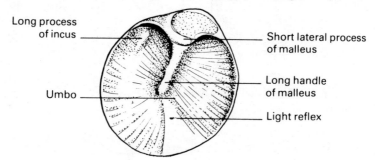

Long process of incus

Short lateral process of malleus

Umbo

Long handle of malleus

Light reflex

Figure 5   The features of the tympanic membrane seen on examination with an auroscope

The malleus articulates with the incus at the head. The incus is shaped like a two-pronged tooth; it has a body, which articulates with the malleus, and both a short and long process. The short process is attached by a ligament to the posterior wall of the middle ear, while the long process runs parallel to the handle of the malleus. The lower end of the long process articulates with the head of the stapes.

The stapes consists of a head, neck and anterior and posterior limbs which both go down to an oval base plate. Figure 4 shows clearly how the stapes really does resemble a stirrup. The base plate fits snugly in the oval window, an important junction between the middle and inner ears.

The tiny joints between these bones are fascinating, that between the malleus and incus being a saddle-shaped joint and that between the incus and stapes being a ball-and-socket joint. In each case, they have an articular capsule and many other features of the big joints of the body.

The two small muscles of the middle ear have already been mentioned – the tensor tympani and the stapedius muscles. The tensor tympani ends in a tiny tendon which is inserted into the upper end of the handle of the malleus. The stapedius also ends in a tendon which is inserted into the neck of the stapes. The two muscles act together and are thought, by their simultaneous contraction, to offer some protection to the delicate structures of the middle ear when they are subjected to very loud sounds. It can be seen that their action would result in a decrease in the vibrations of the middle ear in response to a large auditory stimulus.

The inner ear is situated more medially in the petrous part of the temporal bone and may be divided into two main areas, the cochlea, which is concerned with hearing, and the semicircular canals, which are concerned with balance. However, it is not really possible to divide them as they form one continuous bony structure which surrounds a continuous membranous sac. This is, in fact, a completely closed sac, although it sends out various branches into the complicated shapes of the inner ear. The membranous sac is smaller than the bony structure that surrounds it, and the space between them is filled with fluid known as *perilymph*. The sac itself also contains fluid, known as *endolymph*.

The cochlea, or organ of hearing, has, as we have already implied, a central column, which is cone-shaped and known

as the *modiolus*, surrounded by two-and-a-half turns of a
canal wound round the central core. The appearance of the
cochlea has been likened by some to the shell of a snail.

From the modiolus a spiral lamina of bone extends into the
canal like the thread of a screw. From the outer edge of this
lamina, two membranes extend to the walls of the canal so
that the latter is divided throughout its length into three
chambers. The upper chamber is called the *scala vestibuli*,
the middle chamber between the two membranes is the *scala
media* and the area nearest to the base is the *scala tympani*.
The membrane nearest the apex is known as *Reissner's
membrane* while the other membrane is called the *basilar
membrane*.

The bony cochlea opens into the bony vestibule, and the
oval window leads into this space.

The three semicircular canals – that is, the superior
semicircular canal, the lateral canal and the posterior canal –
are all set at right angles to one another (see Figure 4) and all
three open into the bony vestibule. The reader can now
understand the continuous nature of the two parts of the
inner ear.

The cochlea has a minute bony canal, known as the
aqueduct of the cochlea, which allows the perilymph to
drain into the subarachnoid space. The importance of this in
cases of meningitis and encephalitis can be immediately
realized, as there is a direct route for organisms to the most
important part of the organ of hearing. Hence, as we have
already said, approximately 5% of all cases of meningitis
subsequently develop a profound hearing loss. This is
discussed below in Chapter 12.

Whereas it was thought that, as the membranous sac of
both cochlea and semicircular canals were closed, they provided no drainage system for the endolymph, it is now known
that the endolymph does not remain static. However, the
mechanism of the drainage system is still not known.

It has already been said that the membranous sac of the

inner ear follows the bony shape closely, but, in the bony vestibule, it forms two different parts, the *saccule* and the *utricle*. The membranous cochlea opens into the saccule while the semicircular canals, which are dilated into ampullae at their ends, open into the utricle.

The method by which saccule and utricle are joined is strange but interesting. The saccule sends off a narrow duct called the *ductus endolymphaticus*, while the utricle sends off a fine tube called the *ductus utriculo-saccularis*. It is these two ducts which join, thus causing the whole membranous system to be closed and continuous.

The epithelium of the membranous cochlea is highly specialized and it is here that we find the *organ of Corti* on the basilar membrane with hair cells which are plentifully supplied by the auditory or 8th nerve.

Near the centre of the organ of Corti lies a double row of pillars called the inner and outer rods of Corti. These run along the total length of the scala media and are surrounded by the hair cells, on the inner side a single row, and on the outer side three rows. The outer hair cells are considerably longer than the inner ones; both sets of hair cells are supplied by fibres from the 8th nerve.

From the upper edge of the spiral lamina runs a projecting membrane called the *tectorial membrane* which is so spaced that it projects over the tips of the hair cells and is in close contact with them. The tectorial membrane is only joined near the spiral lamina, the other edge is 'floating' and free to move with the movement of the hair cells.

An elongated *spiral ganglion* is contained within a canal which winds round the central column of the cochlea. The peripheral branches from this ganglion supply the structures mentioned above, in other words, plentiful fibres go to the hair cells while the central branches leave the bone through the internal auditory meatus, thus making up the cochlear portion of the 8th nerve which finally sends fibres to the temporal cortex.

I have called this chapter a physicians' revision of anatomy because it seems to me that only by remembering the structure of the ear does one then remember the pathways of sound through the ear and finally to the temporal lobes of the brain.

For those who are interested in the further auditory pathways, I will add a little more about the final route to the cerebral cortex. The *auditory nerve* consists of the *cochlear division*, concerned with hearing, and the *vestibular division*, arising from the area of the semicircular canals and concerned with balance. I will limit this brief description to the cochlear nerve. The fibres arise from the spiral ganglion, already described, and enter the lower border of the pons. It is very close to the 7th nerve which emerges from the brain in this area, but is separated from it by the vestibular nerve. The fibres then run to the ventral and dorsal cochlear nuclei. From both nuclei, new fibres connect with the dorsal nucleus of the corpus trapezoideum of the same or of the opposite side. Following relay fibres then ascend through the pons and midbrain as the lateral lemniscus to terminate in the *inferior colliculus* and the *medial geniculate body* which are known as the *lower auditory centres*. From here new fibres arise which finally reach the auditory cortex.

From the dorsal nucleus of the corpus trapezoideum, fibres pass to the medial longitudinal bundle which gives access to the nuclei of the 3rd, 4th and 6th cranial nerves. This explains how auditory stimuli can produce reflex movements of the eyes, such as the blink reflex or the auropalpebral reflex.

We can now follow the passage of sound signals from the air to the cerebral cortex where they are interpreted and voluntary responses initiated. Sound waves coming into the external ear, through the external auditory canal, reach the tympanic membrane, a structure which is ideally constructed to pick up the vibrations of sound waves. We have already described how the handle of the malleus is closely associated with the tympanic membrane so that the sound waves are passed on to the malleus. The saddle-shaped joint, with its surrounding joint capsule, means that the waves pass in turn to the incus. Similarly, the ball-and-socket joint between the incus and stapes allows the stapes, and hence the base plate fitting in the oval window, to move in response to sound waves.

Up to this stage, in the healthy middle ear, the vibrations have all been taking place in air. They now move on to a different type of system but one in which the sound waves can still travel very well. The oval window opens into the inner ear, where it will be remembered that the space between the bony and membranous inner ears is filled with fluid, the perilymph. Therefore, at this stage, the sound waves pass from air to fluid. Movement in the fluid produces movement of the delicate hair cells with consequent stimulation of the tiny branches of the 8th nerve.

It is thought that notes of varying frequencies are associated with different groups of cells along the basilar membrane. Various explanations for this have been suggested over the years but to date no theory has fully explained the complex conversion of sound into electrical potential within the cochlea.

In any case, it has been shown that patients having specific high-frequency or low-frequency hearing loss also have specific degeneration in one part of the basilar membrane while the remainder is relatively intact. Also it seems to be generally accepted that high tones are registered in the basal turn of the cochlea.

Chapter 5

WHEN AND WHERE?

Routine hearing checks should start at the age of 7 months. At this age, there appears to be a definite developmental milestone when a baby is able to localize *small* sounds, of 35–40 dB, 1 m from the ear and on a level with the meatus. If tests are done at 6 months, it is very common to find that the child gives perfect results on one side but ambivalent or even very poor results on the other. If the examiner is unaware that this is a common result at 6 months, both he and the parents become very worried. It is not uncommon for such babies to be referred to an audiology clinic. When they reach the clinic, they are usually about 1 month older and the results are perfect. This has meant several weeks of unnecessary anxiety for the parents, so it is therefore very important to begin checks at 7 months. If at this age the test is unsatisfactory, it should be repeated at 8 months. If this remains unchanged, referral to an audiology clinic should be a firm rule. This gives the audiologist time to see the child, either once or twice as appropriate, make moulds and supply hearing aids, which can be in use by the first birthday (see Chapters 13 and 14).

Many doctors, on finding that the 7–8 month tests are unsatisfactory, seem to be unwilling to believe the results of their tests. They find excuses for the results they have seen, for example, 'He's very tired today – he usually has his sleep now', 'I think he's hungry and only interested in his bottle', 'I think he was far too interested in the toy that the other lady was holding', etc. Doctors and parents combine to find an excuse in order to escape the real reason. Parents are only too happy to collude in this exercise, and, if it is not initiated by the doctor, it will almost certainly be initiated by the unhappy parent. I do urge that examiners, having made careful accurate tests, should have faith in their own results and act upon them.

If the 7 month test is satisfactory, the next test of hearing should be at 18 months, the third at 3 years and the fourth at $4\frac{1}{2}$ years. The reader may ask why it is necessary to repeat tests provided the initial ones have been done carefully and precisely. The first and obvious answer is that the child may have had repeated attacks of upper respiratory tract infections since he was last seen, resulting in eustachian catarrh and possibly 'glue ear' with its resultant small hearing loss in the lower frequencies. There seems no doubt that chronic secretory otitis media can be seen in very young babies and there is equally no doubt that parents should know about this (see Chapter 15).

In addition, there are some cases of congenital hearing loss which are not apparent in the earliest years of life. Autosomal dominant deafness is particularly liable to increase with age. This leads to the extremely interesting fact that research in animals has suggested that in many hereditary forms of deafness the damage to the cochlea is not truly congenital but occurs very soon *after* birth. Fraser[1] likens the situation to that of phenylketonuria and this suggests that further work may establish first the cause and then the prevention of postnatal cochlear degeneration.

Lastly, it now seems a well-established fact that cases of deafness due to rubella occasionally tend to increase in severity during the first and even the second years of life.

Thus, we have three very good reasons for testing hearing regularly at the times suggested. The reason for the initial test at 7 months has already been stated. A test at 18 months also enables the examiner to check on whether speech is developing. The normal 18-month-old child has a small, useful vocabulary of nouns and is also using jargon, or long strings of joined sounds, with consonants present and speech intonation and patterns clearly audible.

At 3 years old, the child is using subject–verb–object constructions, and many are already extending these, approaching the stage of complex sentences which should certainly be established by the age of 4 years.

At the same examinations, the stage of verbal comprehension which has been reached should also be checked. The 18-month-old hands common well-known objects, such as cup, spoon and toy car, on request. He also probably begins to respond to the simple domestic commands that he hears every day, such as 'Shut the door', 'Get your shoes', 'Sit down', etc.

The 3-year-old understands commands containing three or four ideas; for example, when using miniature toys he eagerly responds to 'Put mummy on the chair and the baby in the bath', etc. The complexity of his understanding develops very steadily, so that by 4 years he can also understand complex sentences.

Here we should underline the fact that testing hearing at these ages should form part of a general developmental check-up. As it is so obvious that all development is interlinked we recommend that developmental check-ups take place at 7 months, 18 months, 3 years and $4\frac{1}{2}$ years, with intervening examinations whenever they prove necessary for any reason. I have already stated that when a test is failed at 7 months, it should be repeated 1 month later, followed by referral to an audiologist if necessary. A failure at 18 months, 3 years or $4\frac{1}{2}$ years, combined with poor speech development, merits immediate referral. If, however, speech is entirely normal, then the examining doctor can afford to retest in a month, to see, for example, whether a temporary conductive deafness associated with an unusual upper respiratory tract infection has cleared up.

It has been stated above that it is our duty to make sure that all mothers know where to go for these tests. Doctors should familiarize themselves with their own areas as suggested in Chapter 1, and the ideal situation is one where the family doctor is notified by the community health clinic when each child has attended, with a synopsis of findings and suggested referrals. Similarly, when family doctors hold well baby clinics, it would save much time if they notified the local community clinic in the same way. This is particularly easy, of course, when there is a health visitor attachment. In the past, there has been little cooperation between the parties involved, but the aim should be for better communication and cooperative work. Family doctors should recognize the expertise offered in community clinics and the latter should only employ trained doctors who will command such respect.

Reference

1. Fraser, G.R. (1976). *The Causes of Profound Deafness in Childhood*, p. 150. (London: Ballière Tindall)

Chapter 6

SITUATIONS FOR TESTING

Assuming that the family have been successfully persuaded to attend the clinic for the developmental examination, and assuming for the moment only that a good hearing test will take its place alongside the tests for speech, vision, motor function and social and emotional development, we must ensure that the child has a good physical examination at this time.

Wherever the examination takes place, it is necessary to choose the room with as much care as possible or to modify conditions as far as possible so that the testing environment is adequate. First of all, as will be seen from accompanying volumes in this series, rooms should contain 6 m clear space for testing. It is quite useless to measure a room and find it has one dimension of 6 m if that 6 m are cluttered by unnecessary furniture. It is very often possible to remove a lot of clutter from a room with the result that everyone is delighted that someone has at last dared to move it!

Secondly, the room must be as quiet as possible. The telephone should not be allowed to interfere with tests. I have known rooms used that are adjacent to main roads where juggernaut lorries rumble by continuously, rooms next to railway lines, rooms beneath main air traffic lanes, and rooms where nothing except other families, waiting their turn outside for the tests, can be heard. Ingenuity must be used to minimize the hazards of all these situations. It may be possible to change the location of the rooms where the tests are undertaken and then remove a great deal of the unnecessary furniture. If the room is cluttered and the examiner has little space to move around behind the baby, the infant is much more likely to spy him visually and turn out of visual curiosity rather than in response to an auditory stimulus.

It may be possible to change the times of developmental examinations, and someone can be allotted to amuse the children so that the amount of 'patient noise' outside is considerably diminished. This relieves the embarrassment of the mother and irritation of the doctor.

Lastly, it should definitely be stated that, at some time in the future, some of my readers may well be asked to advise on new buildings. At that point, I beg you to remember your colleagues who test hearing. Many rooms are proudly displayed to me as 'soundproofed'. In most cases, this means that some acoustic tiling material has been stuck on the walls. But, in these rooms, you can still give a full report on the telephone conversation in the next room and measure 100 + dB of traffic noise. These well-meaning 'soundproofers' have forgotten the windows and doors. Double glazing and double doors are relatively easy and cheap to include at the time of building, but this becomes more and more difficult as a building ages.

Very few of us are likely to have these ideal conditions but I strongly believe that we should campaign for them as vigorously and vociferously as possible. Of course, it is wrong to say that you cannot test hearing because you do not have ideal conditions. But it is, nevertheless, wrong to make a virtue out of poor working conditions. You must accept what is available while working hard to improve your lot. The problem that arises is that if you are surrounded by ambient noise of 40 dB or much more, you will almost unconsciously raise the levels of your auditory stimuli 'to make up for the difficulties'. So, when you check yourself, you will find you are testing at 50, 55 or 60 dB. Also, of course, the examiner who watches the baby turn towards the traffic sounds and comments favourably on this falls into one of the traps mentioned above. As this is such a common error, I will repeat this warning that traffic noise contains many low-frequency sounds which *deaf* babies hear. In addition, there is a strong vibrotactile element in the noise of heavy traffic so that the infant 'feels' the impact rather than 'hears' it.

Chapter 7

TAKING A HISTORY AND
ITS IMPORTANCE

Having succeeded in getting the family to the quietest
available room in the clinic, the question now arises of
taking a history. It must be stressed that it is most unwise to
think of short-cuts when taking a history in this sort of case.
A carefully recorded history will, time and time again, lead
on, via an accurate examination, to a correct diagnosis at the
first interview. This is, of course, most important as parents
are extremely anxious and want 'an answer' to their un-
certainties as soon as possible. Needless to say, this is not
always possible, but, on the other hand, it is *often* possible.
But it does assume that the examiner is willing to spend a
good deal of time with each child and its parents.

It is sensible to start by enquiring about birth rank,
history of pregnancy, birth and neonatal period. If there is
any suspicious factor here, it may be necessary to make
enquiries at the hospital where the birth took place (see
Chapter 2).

This leads on quite naturally to enquiries about all the
early milestones. In infancy, did the baby turn when his
mother entered the room very quietly behind him and out of
his range of vision? Or did he seem very surprised to see her
as she entered his field of vision? This latter symptom is
commonly reported by parents of deaf babies. Did the baby
show startle reflexes to loud noises or was he entirely

unmoved by even the loudest sounds? (For example, I was once told by a mother that her deaf baby was completely oblivious to the fact that she had dropped a pile of plates behind him.) Normal babies show a lot of *interest* in sound even before they reach the developmental stage of being able to localize accurately. Deaf babies, on the other hand, show a marked difference between their intense interest in visual stimuli and their complete unawareness of auditory stimuli.

Linked with this the examiner should enquire about the baby's vocalizations. It is important to remember that very young babies, even as young as 4 weeks, vocalize. Their most obvious vocalization is their cry, but, when they are fed and comfortable, they also make cooing and gurgling sounds which are quite delightful to anyone who listens. But, on careful listening, it will be noticed that these vocalizations are vowel sounds, or sounds within the lower frequency range. At the age of 3–4 months, these sounds change in the normal infant to 'babble' sounds which contain high-frequency sounds. By the age of 6–7 months, the normal infant is putting strings of babble sounds together so that he can hold a responsive 'conversation' with his family. This change does not occur with the deaf infant and parents often comment spontaneously about the vocalizations of their young babies. Sometimes they notice that a baby is very quiet and this is a most suspicious symptom. When the baby is not the first in the family, it is very common for parents to say that his vocalizations 'don't sound like the others at this age'. Sometimes children with a hearing loss are very noisy, but, when the examiner listens, he can notice the absence of consonants, of tuneful quality and of interesting intonation. The baby, who is obviously trying hard to hear his own vocalizations, may produce loud sounds with a markedly flat intonation.

At this early stage, it is important to ask about milestones in other respects too. A 7-month-old baby who is unresponsive to sound may be unresponsive and retarded in other respects. His motor milestones should be recorded, and his response to suitable play material noted. His general interest in his environment is very important, as is the interaction between the baby and his parents and the baby and the examiner. This is why it is so important that routine hearing tests form part of a general developmental examination.

At a later age, the examiner will want to know about speech itself. Does the child use any words, and, if so, how many? Are words joined, and, again, how many? Are they intelligible outside the family circle, either singly or when joined?

The question of verbal comprehension is very important. It would be very interesting to conduct a poll of the answers given by parents to the question 'Does your child understand any words?' One always waits for the 'inevitable' reply 'Oh, he understands everything'. Of course, parents may well be right in assuming that their children 'understand' but they may be understanding the clues, situational, visual or gestural, that are constantly presented to them and which they have had to learn to use skilfully in the absence of verbal understanding. So it is important to ensure, via one's own observations, whether the child is really understanding words presented without any other clues. It is very interesting to consider our methods of communication with our children. Normally, and quite rightly, we use a basis of words strongly backed up by all the other methods mentioned above. Of course, for the normal child learning to talk at the proper time, these are all essential reinforcers as his vocabulary increases. The deaf child has to learn how to manipulate them, and, indeed, it is very surprising to find how soon a child with a significant hearing loss learns to lip-read. All this means that when taking the history do not be satisfied with the glib reply to questions about verbal comprehension. Ask for examples and then evaluate these, and in later examination, see what *proof* can be obtained.

We have briefly mentioned the question of intelligibility, but this should be stressed again as the child with a mild high-frequency hearing loss may develop quite a lot of speech which is meaningful for him but is unintelligible to everyone else because of the omission of those consonants and consonant blends which he cannot hear.

It is important to enquire about the child's play and hopefully the examination gives you a chance to observe this. There is a fascinating stage at around the age of 1 year when a baby ceases to regard common objects, such as a brush, a cup or a spoon, as *merely* interesting things which he can investigate with his hands, eyes and mouth, bang against another object, such as a table, to produce an interesting noise, and which he can 'cast' or throw to the ground, perhaps hoping that it will be retrieved by the long-suffering adults around him. Around this age, he also begins to understand the symbolic value of these objects and to define them by use. So that, before casting them, he puts the brush to his hair in obvious imitation of his mother's action when she brushes his hair, and he holds the cup the right way round, putting it up to his lips as if to have a drink, while the spoon may be used to 'stir' in the cup. The baby at this stage is demonstrating in play that he realizes the symbolic nature of these objects. At around 18 months, the child brushes a doll's hair and 'gives it a cup of tea'. As the child gets older, this symbolic play becomes more and more complicated until we reach the 3–4-year-old who loves to dress up and act out an imaginary situation drawn from his experience of life (the favourite must be 'Mothers and Fathers'). The normal, but hard-of-hearing, child defines by use in the usual way and also develops symbolic play in the normal way. Although the deaf child may have no expressive language and no verbal comprehension, his ability to symbolize, or his 'inner language', is intact. This is very important in differential diagnosis, say, between the child

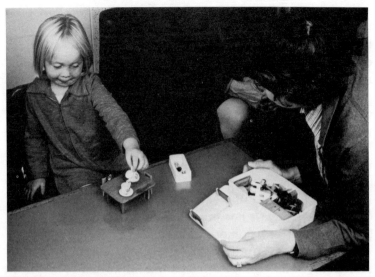

Figure 6   A child with a mild autosomal dominant hearing
loss showing normal symbolic play at 3 years of age

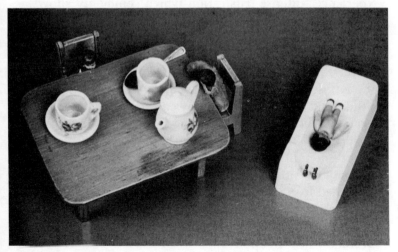

Figure 7   Close-up picture of the spontaneous arrangement
made by the child in Figure 6. Toys were handed randomly

who does not talk because he is deaf and the child who does not talk because he is retarded. The latter shows similar retardation in his 'inner language'. With such a child, definition by use of common objects is not to be seen until a much later age. The young retarded child is also unaware of the symbolic value of miniature toys and, therefore, continues to mouth them, cast them or pile them up meaninglessly. The young deaf child, on the other hand, uses such toys to make a meaningful arrangement, often using gesture or mime as he does so.

If the child is not communicating by speech, it is important for the examiner to ask what method of communication he is using. Is he taking his mother to what he wants? Does he point or use more complicated gesture, or does he mime? The older, undiagnosed deaf child will use the most interesting and complicated mime in order to try to overcome the frustration of inability to communicate.

This leads the examiner on to asking the parents about the child's behaviour. The child who cannot communicate often experiences intense frustration which commonly shows as temper tantrums. As the treatment of a deaf child progresses, so the tantrums lessen. On the other hand, the child with communication problems may choose the other path and retreat into himself. I well remember seeing a 4-year-old girl whose speech was poor and who was intensely withdrawn. Investigation showed her to have a high-frequency hearing loss combined with a difficult social background. It was little wonder that she had given up most of her attempts to communicate in such a harsh and unpromising situation. This child was under a psychiatrist who failed to realize the significance of her hearing loss. In fact, it is not uncommon for children whose hearing loss has not been diagnosed to be referred to departments of child psychiatry (see Chapter 3).

Chapter 8

METHODS OF TESTING HEARING: (a) DISTRACTION TECHNIQUES

There are three main clinical methods of testing hearing:

(1) Distraction tests.
(2) Cooperative tests using speech.
(3) Conditioning tests which do not depend on speech.

The first category is described in this chapter.

DISTRACTION TESTS

Distraction tests are used from the age of 7 months, and, as already indicated in Chapter 5, they do not give reliable results before this age. In fact, they can show misleading and ambivalent results which give concern to all. What then can be done before the age of 7 months when parents bring their baby with anxieties about its hearing? The first answer is to take a careful history which, as already seen, can give a multitude of clues. The next step is to take a very careful look at the whole of the baby's development to date. If it is obvious from this that the whole of development is retarded, then it is possible that poor hearing responses form a part of this. The baby's own vocalizations should be carefully noted. Failure to hear any vocalizations except crying throughout a long and careful examination is suspicious. If, after 4 months, vocalizations do not contain any high-frequency sounds, again this is suspicious. The most useful clinical tool to use before the age of 6–9 months is a very small bell. A normal neonate shows a very marked startle reflex, and a normal baby of 6 weeks will, very probably, show some reaction to a much smaller sound, that is to a small bell rung 15 to 22 cm from the meatus. The most usual reaction is 'stilling', that is, all the baby's small movements cease, quite perceptibly, for a moment. There may also be eye-widening or eye-turning towards the sound source. Occasionally, there is a slow movement of the whole head towards the sound source. These tiny indications increase as the infant gets older. Incidentally, this very young age is the *only* one at which it is permissible to use a bell in screening tests.

A 6-week-old infant, who is not actively hungry or uncomfortable, can be soothed by the sound of his mother's voice and, again, this increases as the infant gets older. The 'feel' of the parents about the baby's hearing is extremely important, and if parents say they think the baby is deaf they are only ignored at your peril. They should always be taken seriously and it is usually preferable to refer them to an audiology centre straight away.

There is one electrodiagnostic test, the *crossed acoustic response* screening test of hearing, which, being totally non-invasive, is particularly suitable for very young babies and is available at several centres now. This test is discussed, with others, in Chapter 17. The usual procedure is to do the test and then discuss the results with the parents, giving them at least some indication of whether your results confirm or contradict their anxieties. It is then explained to them that it is necessary to wait for further clinical tests at the age of 7 months in order to confirm the diagnosis fully. If it seems likely that the infant has a hearing loss, the family should be put in touch with the peripatetic teaching service and the family doctor and health visitor should be advised, for such a family is often left in an agonizing suspense of indecision. If they can have every opportunity to discuss their predicament and be given useful advice about the earliest forms of auditory training, in which they are involved, this can at least alleviate the situation to some extent. It should also be explained that, in any case, amplification is only rarely used before the age of 7 months, and that what they are doing for their baby is the appropriate treatment for one so young.

Distraction tests are used between the ages of 7 months and $1\frac{1}{2}$–2 years. These are the tests that look so 'easy'. Too often they are dismissed in a most casual way – 'anyone can shake a rattle'. In the accurate practice of audiology, these tests are extremely precise and require much practice before the tester can consider himself proficient. Let us first consider the apparatus used. It is, I suppose, the fact that the apparatus is so simple that deludes the unwary into thinking casually about the way in which it is used. The apparatus consists of:

(1) An ordinary china cup and a teaspoon.
(2) Either a Nuffield rattle* or a Manchester rattle †.
(3) The examiner's voice.

Some authorities have ceased to use a cup and spoon but I find it a very useful tool provided one is aware of its limitations. The main criticism of its use is that the examiner is not sure what frequencies are being tested. This is, of course, quite true, but we know, and the physicists can show us, that we are testing across a wide range of frequencies and it does include some low frequencies which

---

* The Nuffield rattle is included in the Stycar apparatus, devised by Dr Mary Sheridan and obtainable from NFER (see Appendix 1).

† The Manchester rattle is obtainable from the Department of Audiology at Manchester University.

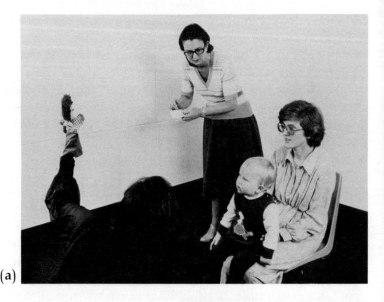

(a)

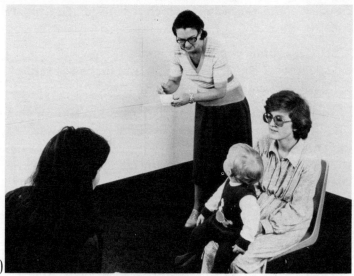

(b)

Figure 8   Use of cup and spoon. (a) One-year-old infant's attention is held by visual stimulus, (b) visual stimulus removed, infant turns briskly to auditory stimulus

are very useful. In addition, it is a familiar homely sound, quite attractive to a baby. When using it, we *stroke* the bowl of the spoon along the rim of the cup to produce a sound of around 35–40 dB. The rim of the cup should *never* be tapped. Once a tapping sound is produced, an acceptable screening level of 40 dB has been exceeded. It is specially necessary to be careful to avoid an initial *tap* when commencing the test. I am afraid that this test is, all too commonly, misused. Many doctors and health visitors tap away, without caution, at 60 dB (or more) and consequently many babies with a partial hearing loss slip through the net until they fail to talk at the expected time, when they are referred to a specialized clinic because of 'a speech problem'. (NB It *is* possible to produce 90–100 dB of sound by tapping a cup vigorously before you finally shatter it. It is essential to remember that tapping the cup *in any way* produces an invalid screening test!)

The second piece of apparatus used is a rattle, but it must be either a Nuffield or a Manchester rattle. Both these rattles produce high-frequency sounds of around 8 kHz without any low-frequency components. Thus we have a specific test for high-frequency hearing. But, alas, one finds only too often that ordinary play rattles are used and, again, are being shaken without any thought given to the decibels produced. Many of the common play rattles produce 70–80 dB with an almost minimum shake. After all, their function is to produce an *easily* heard noise which will attract babies from 4 months onwards. They certainly do not measure the threshold of high-frequency hearing in a 7-month-old. The Manchester rattle should not be shaken for it can produce levels up to 65 dB. But, if it is gently turned from side to side, it produces the required level of 35–40 dB assuring all the other precautions are observed (see below, page 71). The Nuffield rattle should be held like a pen and used as if stirring a cup of coffee. This, too, produces 35–40 dB when all the test precautions are observed. When examiners are presented with any other kind of rattle, they will be doing parents and

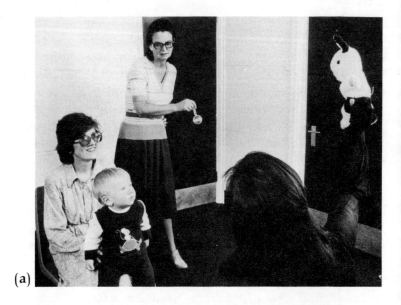

(a)

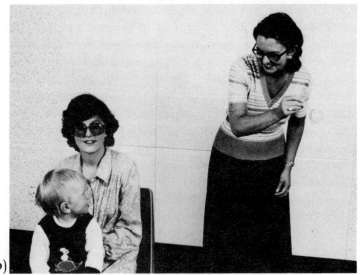

(b)

Figure 9   Use of Manchester rattle. (a) One-year-old infants attention obtained by visual stimulus, (b) visual stimulus removed, brisk turn to auditory stimulus

infants a great service if they remove the offending article and see that, in future, it is only used as its manufacturer intended, a plaything to be handled by the baby only.

The third piece of apparatus required is the simplest and is, of course, the examiner's voice. He should use this to produce a high-frequency sound, a low-frequency sound and also very briefly, in a conversational manner. The high-frequency sound usually chosen is the sound *ss-ss-ss-ss* said several times in quick and rapid sequence very softly. This sound is at the highest end of the frequencies used in speech. A convenient low frequency sound is *oo-oo-oo* used in a sing-song manner. This can quite conveniently be joined with the child's name and should be followed by a few convers-ational phrases said in a very soft voice, such as 'See what I've got, John' (showing toy, etc.) or 'Can you find me, John?' (smiling). This little scrap of conversation is import-ant for, after all, we want to know the child's ability to respond to speech in general, as well as measuring his response to distinct frequencies. The examiner must not fall into the trap of using whispered conversation as this involves mainly the high frequencies and we have already tested these. He should aim at putting some laryngeal tone into his voice but keeping it below 40 dB. This is, in fact, something that requires a good deal of practice.

Just as the tools must be used very precisely, so the situation of the hearing test must be set up very precisely. The mother or mother substitute should sit upright on a straight-backed chair facing the first examiner. The baby should sit on her lap also facing the first examiner who is immediately in front of but a few metres away from him. The mother should make sure that the baby is sitting quite straight, firmly supported but not leaning back against her. The role of the first examiner is to keep the baby's attention straight in front of him, and, for this purpose, he normally uses a variety of toys which will interest the baby and keep him looking forward until the first examiner is aware that the second examiner is in position and ready to start giving the auditory stimuli. When the baby is 7 months, the second examiner should be standing 1 m away from the baby, just behind him so that he is completely out of the baby's field of vision. It is important for the examiner to remember how wide the field of vision is and beware of giving the infant a whole series of visual clues with the cup, the rattle and his own head! With the two examiners working as a team, the first examiner removes the visual stimulus, and, at that moment, the second examiner gives the auditory stimulus. The normally hearing 7-month-old baby is very inquisitive and turns briskly to investigate the sound. *All the sounds, with the exception of the Nuffield rattle, should be given at 1 m from the baby's ear and on a level with the meatus*, and repeated, of course, on both right and left sides. The Nuffield rattle must be used 22–30 cm from the ears, but this is the only exception to the 1 m rule. The examiners must beware of giving other clues to the baby, such as reflections or even squeaky shoes.

The first examiner must be very wary of producing a visual stimulus so fascinating that the baby ignores the auditory stimuli. It is best for two people to learn to work together as a team. They will then learn what sort of visual stimulus is useful for each age group between 7 months and 2 years. The 7-month-old baby only needs the mildest of visual stimuli (a ball on a string, for instance) to persuade him to look straight forward. In fact, he may become so interested in the first examiner's face that it is necessary for the latter to move gently away so that the auditory stimulus can be given to best advantage. However, as the baby gets older, he wishes to look around him, wriggle off his mother's knee and reach out for the visual stimulus. It then becomes a very skilful procedure to keep him still with his eyes and interest in front of him on something the first examiner is doing that can be gradually moved out of sight (puppets are very useful here) so that the second examiner can produce the auditory stimulus at an absolutely crucial moment.

There are, of course, some examiners who are not able to work as a team, although this is strongly recommended whenever two people can learn the skills together. In the case of a lone practitioner, he has to depend upon a picture or toy placed in front of the child, but out of reach, to act as a visual stimulus. A picture on a wall is probably the better of what are really poor substitutes, as an active child merely leans forwards and wriggles in an effort to reach a toy of interest.

In summary, if the examiner uses the right tools, in the right way, with the conditions of testing scrupulously observed, he can test both low and high frequencies and also hearing for speech at 35–40 dB. This is the aim of the

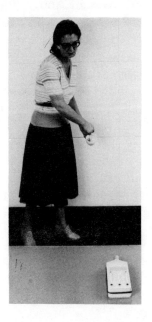

Figure 10   Checking level of sound used with a Dawe sound level meter. The cup and spoon were 1 m away from and level with the meter

examination, but these are precise tests and precise conditions must be observed.

If a sound level meter is available, the examiner should constantly recheck his performance to make sure that his standards are being maintained. If this is not possible, then colleagues should advise one another on their performances.

So far we have talked about the 7-month-old baby for whom all tests are given at meatus level. When the baby reaches the age of 9 months, however, his localization abilities have improved. He is now able to hear the same small sounds, of 35–40 dB, at a distance of 1 m but both below and above meatus level. It is, in fact, best to give the test at meatus level first in the older baby. If this is successful, the examiner can proceed to testing the baby's ability to localize below and above meatus level. The 9-month-old baby, for example, who shows some general mild immaturity may still only localize at meatus level.

In all the tests described, only definite turns of the head are an acceptable 'pass'. Stilling or eye-movements should be noted but *not* accepted as proof of hearing. In the absence of a completely satisfactory test using all the described methods, it should be repeated again in 1 month. If it remains unsatisfactory then, as already stated in Chapter 5, it is essential to seek further help. It is at this time that the examiner must avoid the pitfalls already mentioned of finding excuses for the failure. He must bravely show faith in his tests and refer appropriately.

Chapter 9

METHODS OF TESTING HEARING:
(b) COOPERATIVE TESTS INVOLVING SPEECH
(c) CONDITIONING TECHNIQUES

COOPERATIVE TESTS INVOLVING SPEECH

After the child has reached the age of 18 months to 2 years, he recognizes the simple auditory stimuli that have been used, so does not bother to verify his auditory information with visual information. In other words, he does not bother to turn to these stimuli. It is at this time that other methods which are both interesting to the child and accurate for the examiner must be found.

For the child who is developing some comprehension of speech, there is a selection of tests using toys and pictures appropriate for the various age groups. This chapter merely describes some tests which have been found very useful in the author's clinic and many other community health clinics in the London area. A list of apparatus available for other tests is given in Appendix 1.

At about 18 months to 2 years, the child is developing a very useful naming vocabulary. Thus, a small selection of

75

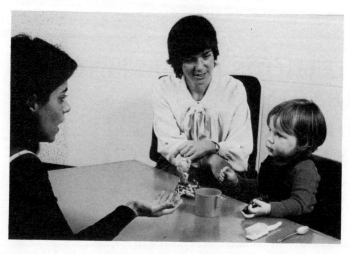

Figure 11   An intelligent 18-month-old child attempting a five-toy test

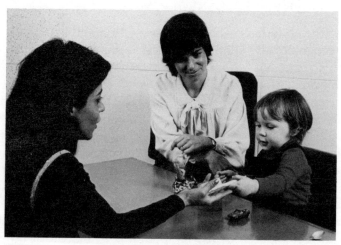

Figure 12   The test in Figure 11 proceeding well. Note that the examiner remains close to this very young child to maintain rapport

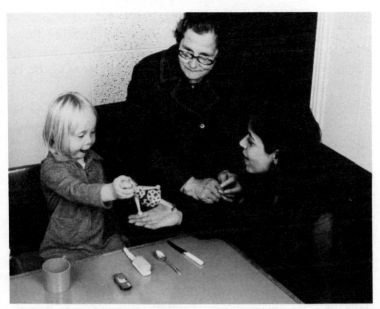

Figure 13 A 3-year-old child with mild autosomal dominant hearing loss attempting the same five-toy test as shown
in Figures 11 and 12

toys with familiar names make a very useful start to this type
of test. The bright 18-month-old and the normal 2-year-old
recognize the names for a cup, spoon, toy car, doll and
brush. In this very first toy test, the toys are presented to the
child one at a time and each is named by the examiner at
conversation distance using a firm clear voice (Figures 11
and 12). When all the toys are placed in front of the child, he
is then asked by the examiner to give them to him, one at a
time, with the examiner still at conversation distance and
still using a clear firm voice. As the child hands each one, the
examiner thanks him, praises him, and replaces it on the
table in a slightly different position in the line of toys. This
stage of the test is of vital importance as it tells the examiner
whether or not the child has sufficient vocabulary to
undertake this kind of test. (It is remarkable how many

examiners omit this stage, assume that the child is familiar with the words, and proceed to a useless 'hearing test'.) Having satisfied himself that he can proceed, the examiner explains to the child that he is going to do the game again. He then does three things:

(1) He covers his mouth, as lip-reading starts at an incredibly young age.

(2) He lowers his voice.

(3) He moves very gently away from the child. If he retreats 3 m away at once, he will lose the attention of the very young child. He is only moving away in order to deliver a voice of 40 dB at the child's ear. He then asks the child, once again, either to show him each toy in turn or else to 'give it to Mummy'.

The extremely important part of this test is that the examiner should be aware of whether or not he is using a 40 dB voice. It is unlikely that most examiners will have access to a sound level meter, but, if they do at any time, they should take the opportunity of practising the levels of their own voice. It is essential to be aware of the volume of your own voice that approximates to 40 dB and, in a similar way, very useful to know the volume that approximates to 60 dB. In this way, you learn the approximate change in your voice that is equivalent to a 20 dB increase or decrease. In the same way, you can practise the levels of your voice at varying distances from the test subject. If no sound level meter is available, the tester and his partner should practise together in a quiet room. An adult with normal hearing should stand 3 m away from the tester, who should then practise a voice which his partner can only *just* hear without total discrimination of the words used. If this same volume of voice is then used about 1 m from the child, an approximation to 40 dB is achieved[1]. Again, it must be stressed that this is a technique requiring much practice and all the toy tests that we use depend absolutely upon the correct level of voice being used.

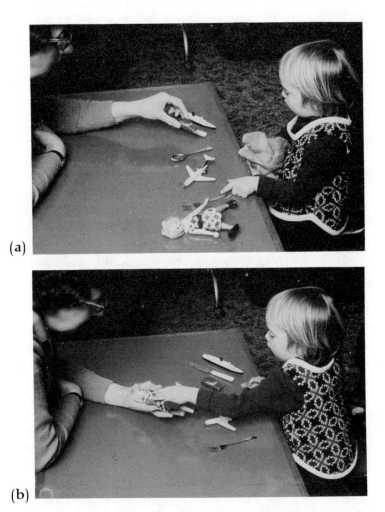

(a)

(b)

Figure 14 A 3-year-old child doing Sheridan's seven-toy test. (a) The examiner is naming the toys. (b) The child hands back the toys on request, proving that she is familiar with the words to be used for testing her hearing

As the child gets older, the number of toys used in the test can be increased, so that, from the age of 3 years onwards, Dr Mary Sheridan's seven-toy test[2] with doll, ship, aeroplane, car, knife, fork and spoon – is extremely useful. The method is the same as described for the simpler test using only five toys. The age at which a child can attempt this test varies depending upon his intelligence and background (for instance, many London children are unfamiliar with a ship). The precautions already described must be observed. The mouth must be covered to prevent lip-reading and the voice reaching the child must be around 40 dB and not more. The actual distance at which the examiner stands from the child is not crucial as long as the examiner is aware of how to modulate the volume of his voice. This point is important as many children lose rapport or interest and move from the table if the examiner is too far away from him and especially if he moves too far too quickly. If the child is older, however, ears may be tested separately and the examiner may move to each side confidently.

Again, it is important not to whisper as a whispered voice cuts down the low-frequency sounds and the test is then made into a high-frequency test only. You may, in fact, wish to use such a test under special circumstances, but, at the moment, we are dealing with general screening tests.

This then leads us on to high-frequency screening tests for children. The best and simplest of these, in my view, were devised by Dr Mary Sheridan, and, in addition to these, Barry McCormick has recently introduced another interesting and easily used test for children over a wide range of different ages.

Dr Sheridan used two sets of pictures. The first set of six provides a test for the 3-year-old, although once again the age of use varies considerably with the particular child under test. The six pictures are ship, seat, feet, chick, pig, and fish. The reader can see at once that the names of the pictures all contain high-frequency sounds – *sh, s, f* and *ch*.

The child with a high-frequency loss hearing the same vowels paired with different high-frequency consonants makes the expected mistakes, for example, he hears *feet* instead of *seat*, or vice versa, *ship* instead of *chick*, etc. Such mistakes are strongly indicative of a high-frequency loss and should *always* be investigated further.

The method of administering the test is exactly the same as that described for the toy tests. The three rules should again be remembered, and, I think, bear restating:

(1) The pictures should be named for the child, using a loud firm voice.

(2) Remaining at conversation distance, the child should be asked to point out the pictures, one by one. This is to ensure that he is fully familiar with the names of the objects in the picture. (Once again, it is surprising how many examiners omit this stage, thus invalidating the test completely.)

(3) If the child is familiar with the names, the examiner covers his lips, lowers his voice and retreats gently from the child, judging how far he can go without losing the child's interest and cooperation. Once again, the difficult part for the examiner is to judge the volume of his voice so that he is delivering 40 dB at the child's ear. Again, it is best if the examiner starts with a 'voiced voice', especially if this is being used as the main screening test in a development check. However, if it is being used as part of an examination for a well-suspected high-frequency loss, the use of a whispered voice may be a useful addition to a battery of tests.

When the child is older, around 4 years but again varying very much with the child's background and environment, the twelve high-frequency picture test may be used. This is simply a more complicated version of the six high-frequency picture test. The pictures used are seat, feet, teeth, fish, dish, tree, key, leaf, wheel, pig, ship, and chick. The method of using the test is as previously described, but of course with an older child there are many more opportunities to demonstrate how he can hear the vowels, that is, low-frequency sounds, but consistently muddle the consonants, or the high-frequency sounds. Provided all the precautions are meticulously observed, this can be a very useful diagnostic tool. However, as with all these tests that appear so 'easy', if the method of administration is not accurate, the diagnosis may be missed. Again, it is the tester rather than the test that is inadequate.

Barry McCormick has devised a test* which is very similar in principle to Mary Sheridan's. He uses pairs of toys which have a common vowel but different consonants in their names, that is, cup and duck, plate and plane, shoe and spoon, house and cow, horse and fork, lamb and man, and key and tree. The method of administration is exactly similar and it has two advantages. Firstly, the number of pairs needed can be varied according to the age and/or intelligence of the child, and, secondly, the use of actual toys probably increases the interest value to the child.

There are, of course, other similar tests but all depend upon similar principles, and if the reader has a favourite, for instance The Kendall Toy Test or the Reed RNID Hearing Test Cards, which have not been mentioned through lack of space, he should examine his own methods of delivery very critically and be sure that all the precautions mentioned above are being observed.

CONDITIONING TESTS OF HEARING

The tests discussed in the last section are very useful for the

---

* The apparatus is available from Barry McCormick, Institute of Sound and Vibration Research, The University, Southampton SO9 5NH.

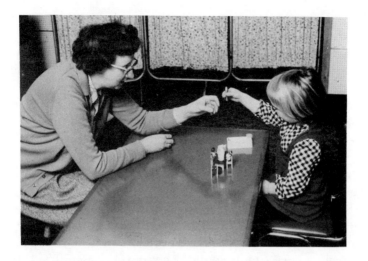

Figure 15   After hearing tests, symbolic play or 'inner language' is tested

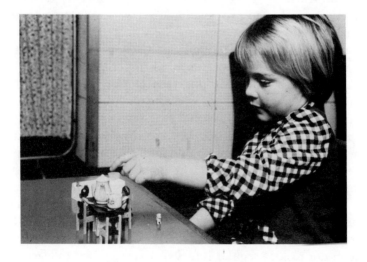

Figure 16   The obvious enjoyment of a 3-year-old demonstrating normal symbolic play

child who is developing speech but useless for the child who presents to us without any speech or any understanding of speech. This is usually the crux of the whole matter. 'Why is my child not talking?' 'Is he deaf?' 'Is he retarded?' 'Has he a specific language problem?' And so on. We have already said that distraction tests cease to be useful at around the age of 2 years. So it is necessary to have tests which require no speech, retain a child's interest and measure hearing with a reasonable degree of accuracy. Simple conditioning tests fulfil these criteria and can be understood by children with a mental age of $2\frac{1}{2}$ years.

Such tests are based on the fact that it is possible to teach a child with normal hearing to perform a simple motor task, such as put a brick in a box or a pegman in a boat, every time he hears a very simple sound. The sound chosen first is the word *go*, in other words every time the examiner says the word *go*, the child puts a brick in a box or performs a similar simple motor task. There are obvious advantages in choosing the word *go*. It is a word that is commonly used in play ('ready, steady, go', for example), it is a simple command that is understood at an early stage of verbal comprehension, and, lastly, it is a suitable low-frequency sound, so the examiner is aware that he is testing for low-frequency hearing. If the child is unaware of the meaning of the sound, it is immaterial as far as the usefulness of the test is concerned.

At first, the child's parents are involved in the game, then, when the child has shown interest, he is helped to put the brick in the box at the right moment. It is important that time should be taken over these early stages so that the child is thoroughly familiar with the procedure. It is also important that the auditory stimulus is not given at regular repeated intervals or the child will simply carry on repeating the motor task at regular intervals having failed to learn the real connection between stimulus and response. When the child has learned absolutely reliably to respond to the stimulus, then the examiner ensures that he removes the visual clue, by covering his mouth and/or going behind the child. At this stage, the examiner is testing the child's ability to respond to a known and practised task but any response is now going to be to an auditory stimulus only. It is therefore essential to start with a *loud* auditory stimulus. Following this, the examiner gradually lowers his voice until the responses cease. In this way, with only the simplest of apparatus and the expenditure of a reasonable amount of time, the examiner obtains extremely useful information about the child's low-frequency hearing. But, as with other tests, the onus is on the examiner to observe accuracy and not allow the very simplicity of the procedure to let him drift into small inaccuracies which invalidate the test. This test, as with the others previously described, can be used binaurally or with separate ears. It can be used with the examiner quite close to a timid and apprehensive child or a child who dances away from his seat the moment the examiner moves away from him. Or, with a cooperative and interested child, it may be used several metres away from each ear. (Once again, it is important for the tester to know the volume of the voice that he is using (see p. 78)). In practice, children usually enjoy this test very much and it is not unusual to see them doing it again with mother or sibling at the end of the examination.

A similar test for high-frequency hearing may be made by substituting the sound *sss* for the word *go*. In this case the child would be instructed that every time he hears the sound *sss* ('like a snake'), he is to put a brick in the box, pegman in the boat, etc. If, as would be wise, he has already performed the low-frequency test, he will be totally familiar with the proceedings. If not, explanations are given and precautions observed exactly as before. Once again, with minimal apparatus, a very reasonable idea of high-frequency hearing can be obtained.

In each of these tests, there is no doubt that the examiner who is screening hearing is left with the knowledge of whether or not his patient requires further examination from someone specializing in the testing of hearing in children, a developmental paediatrician or a paediatric neurologist – or ideally all three in a team effort.

THE USE OF THE AUDIOMETER

Simple conditioning tests, as described in the last section, are a good preparation for the use of an audiometer, whether the *free field audiometer* or the *pure tone audiometer* with headphones.

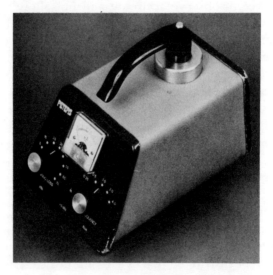

Figure 17   The free field audiometer

The free field audiometer is being used more and more in primary clinics and is a small machine (see Figure 17) which produces pure tones at 250 Hz, 500 Hz, 1000 Hz (1 kHz), 2000 Hz (2 kHz) and 4000 Hz (4 kHz). Each frequency can be played at a required volume, simply by adjusting two knobs. 250 Hz can be played at 5 dB, 15 dB, 25 dB, 35 dB, 45 dB, 55 dB and 65 dB. On most machines, there is also a small knob which, when pushed, adds an extra 5 dB to the volume. Thus at 250 Hz, it also provides 10 dB, 20 dB, 30 dB, 40 dB, 50 dB, 60 dB and 70 dB. At 500 Hz, 1 kHz, 2 kHz and 4 kHz, the machine, by using all three knobs in conjunction, can produce 5 dB, 10 dB, 15 dB, 20 dB, 25 dB, 30 dB, 35 dB, 40 dB, 45 dB, 50 dB, 55 dB, 60 dB, 65 dB, 70 dB, 75 dB and 80 dB. Note that the machine only produces up to 70 dB at 250 Hz but up to 80 dB at all other frequencies.

This machine produces *pure* tones, that is sounds without any overtones, which, therefore, to the average ear are far less interesting than the complicated everyday sounds that we hear around us and which continually provoke our curiosity and interest.

The free field audiometer may be used in two ways. In children over the age of 1 year but under the *mental* age of 3 years, it can be used as a very useful extra means of distraction in the early distraction tests, in other words, it can be added to the cup and spoon, the rattle and the voice. What is more, if held correctly at 1 m from the meatus, it can give quite an accurate measurement of hearing at all frequencies on both sides. But words of warning must be added immediately. First of all, it should not be used for babies below the age of 1 year. It has been shown quite conclusively that the threshold at which babies below this age turn to pure tones is considerably higher than that at which they turn to the sounds already described which have an interest value. Thus, if the instrument is used for screening tests below the age of 1 year, the test results can be misleading. The same precaution applies to mentally retarded children who often fail to show any interest in pure tones. Lastly, the examiner must be sure to use the instrument at the prescribed distance from the ears. If it is held closer, the volume of sound producing, or not producing, a response must be checked on a sound level meter, because of the Inverse Square Law; this means that the volume of sound at the ear is very greatly affected by moving the machine. All common free field audiometers are calibrated to be held 1 m from the ear.

Probably the greatest use of the machine is with a conditioning technique like that previously described with the simpler play methods using low and high-frequency sounds made by the voice. The method is similar and is, in fact, a very popular game with children having a mental age of 3 years or thereabouts. To recapitulate, the child is taught that every time he hears a sound he makes some simple motor response, such as putting a brick in a box. An ingenious examiner can devise many simple motor responses, and it is often wise to have a variety of play responses available so that the child's interest can be maintained.

At first, the adults or older siblings accompanying the child are taught the procedure and then, when the child begins to show interest, he is helped to do it himself. Finally,

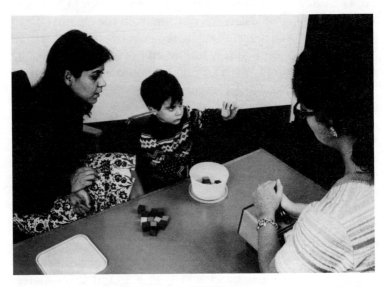

Figure 18   Teaching the conditioning process using the free field audiometer

he is allowed to do it alone. It is generally sensible to start by letting the child see the examiner push the knob that produces the sound. So, at this stage, the child is responding to both visual and auditory stimuli. When the conditioning process has been reliably established, the visual stimulus is removed, by covering the knob with the examiner's hand (Figure 19). The severely deaf child, of course, will then fail to respond as he has been relying totally upon the visual stimulus. In any case, when the visual stimulus is removed, the examiner should always start with the loudest auditory stimulus possible, particularly if there have been some hints already that the child has a hearing loss.

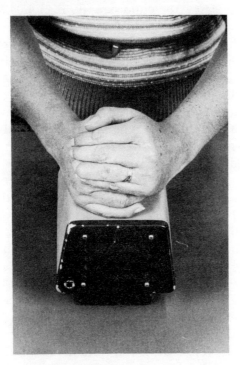

Figure 19   Hiding the visual stimulus when using the free field audiometer

It is very important to make quite sure that the child really is being conditioned to the auditory stimulus, particularly when the suspected loss is great. A very deaf child, always on the lookout for any other sort of clue to help him interpret a situation, may become conditioned to a most extraordinary selection of actions. First of all, he watches the hand that was previously seen to be pressing the knob, and, although now covered, he is alert to the slightest alteration in position of the fingers. The examiner may, without being aware of it, look up at the child whenever he makes the hidden signal. Similarly, he may smile as he presses the knob or even raise his eyebrows, shift his position in his seat etc., and, in these cases, the child happily responds to what, to him, is a regular signal. This is far more likely to happen when the auditory signals are given in a regular rhythm, so, as mentioned previously, they should always be given at irregular intervals. Thus, the reader can see that there are many pitfalls to avoid before one is sure that the child is truly conditioned to an auditory stimulus – and *to no other*.

If the examiner already suspects that the child has a very serious loss, it is likely that the child hears none of the signals produced by the free field audiometer. In this case, it is not only useless to try to use this for conditioning but is bound to be misleading. The child does not understand what is expected of him and either gives completely random responses or chooses another stimulus being unwittingly given to him by an inexperienced examiner. In such cases, it is wise to omit the use of the free field audiometer.

Most very deaf children respond to the loud vibrotactile sound of a drum at about 100 dB and this can be conveniently used to teach the conditioning technique. The fact that the loud sound of a drum contains a vibrotactile element is, in this case, very useful, as it certainly helps the very deaf child to be aware of 'a noise'. In addition, the drum is attractive to the very deaf child who likes to play with it himself as a reward for a successfully completed test.

Once again, the method remains unchanged. At first the child is allowed to see the examiner while he bangs the drum at maximum volume. Mother, father and any brothers or sisters who are present are asked to respond to the drum beat in one of the usual ways, such as putting a brick in the box, etc. The whole thing, as before, is made into a family game and when the patient shows some enthusiasm for taking part he is helped by one of the family to do it correctly. An intelligent 3-year-old soon shows that he needs no help and often pushes away the helping hand so that he is performing independently. The examiner, having got him reliably to this stage, slowly moves to the side, and, finally, behind him. At first the child looks behind to find the examiner, but he can usually soon be persuaded to look in front of him while the examiner produces the loud vibrotactile auditory stimulus behind him. A child who has performed perfectly when the examiner was in front of him, but fails to respond or hesitates when the visual element disappears, should make the examiner very suspicious of a profound hearing loss.

In these ways, by using the free field audiometer or the drum, the examiner can measure, at least to some extent, anything from a very mild conductive hearing loss to a profound sensorineural loss. The free field audiometer may be used binaurally, with the examiner and machine sitting 1 m in front of the child. If the machine is used at a different distance from the child then, once again, the sound levels produced should be checked on a sound level meter. As, in practice, it is unlikely that primary screening clinics will have a sound level meter, it is obviously necessary for most people to test at the accurate distance of 1 m.

If you wish to test each ear separately, this may be attempted by standing at the side of the child, 1 m away from him, with a partner to occlude the opposite ear.

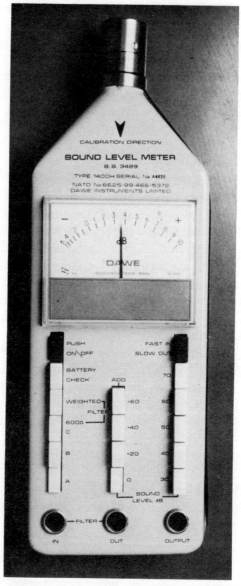

Figure 20   A sound level meter, to check voice or any other
auditory stimulus being used

The examiner has now provided himself with a good deal of information and has also thoroughly prepared the ground for the use of the pure tone audiometer.

References

1. McCormick, B. (1977). The toy discrimination test: an aid for screening the hearing of children above a mental age of two years. *Public Health*, **91**, 67–69
2. Sheridan, M.D. (1976). *Manual for the Stycar Hearing Tests*, 2nd Edn. (Windsor: NFER Publishing Company)

Chapter 10

USE OF THE PURE TONE AUDIOMETER

Whereas previously the use of the pure tone audiometer was limited to very specialized departments and clinics, more and more people are now using them. For example, in London selected school nurses are trained in its use and provided with portable audiometers which they take to schools to do sweep tests. The ages chosen for the sweep tests vary a little from one area to another but are often around 5 and 8 years. The pass limit also varies a little, but 30 dB at frequencies 250 Hz, 500 Hz, 1 kHz, 2 kHz and 4 kHz is usually considered satisfactory. While in specialized departments, 20 dB is considered the lower limit of normal, the extra 10 dB is added for school tests because of the enormous amount of extraneous noise. Although individual schools are usually most helpful, for instance they might remove the percussion band from the classroom next door, sounds from outside the school cannot be eliminated so easily.

In order to help minimize outside sounds, the headphones of the audiometer can be provided with muffs which are a considerable help; now that efficient muffs are available, school screening tests should not be done without them. The main purpose of the school audiometric test is to act as a further screen, and this often produces two distinct categories of children. First, there are those with a sensorineural loss who have not previously been discovered. This may

reflect upon the family or more seriously upon the technique of previous screening tests. Occasionally, of course,
the child has had measles or mumps and a subsequent
unilateral hearing loss passed unnoticed. Secondly, and
much more commonly, the test reveals those children who
have a small, but significant, conductive hearing loss. This is
a cause for concern and usually needs active treatment (see
Chapter 15).

Children who fail a school screening test are referred to a
specialized clinic where a full audiogram and clinical
examination can be carried out.

These school screening tests are, obviously, very important. Even small hearing losses can have a significant effect
upon educational achievement. Therefore, as with training
for screening younger children, the training of personnel
who use pure tone audiometers is very important. Unfortunately it is not uncommon to find mistakes due to
incompetent use of audiometric screening. I am, at the
moment, looking after a small boy who has a moderate
sensorineural hearing loss requiring the use of two postaural
hearing aids. His school medical record indicates that he
'passed' such a screening test at around the age of 5 years. He
was brought to me shortly after this by his mother who felt
that his speech was not as good as it should be. She was, of
course, quite right, but it took me a very long time to
demonstrate to her the reason for this and persuade her that
my results were the correct results. Obviously, she would
have preferred to believe the 'wrong' result and thus remove
the necessity for the use of two hearing aids. This child is
very intelligent, but, if we had failed to diagnose his
moderate hearing loss, he would certainly not have had the
optimal opportunities for benefitting from his education.
This example has been given to indicate the degree of
responsibility that rests upon the shoulders of those who
undertake school screening tests.

Training, again, varies from one area to another. When

school nurses are seconded to my department for training, I feel that it should be divided into three parts. First, the trainee should have ample opportunity to watch the clinics, so she can see the earlier screening tests and begin to appreciate the fact that our simple apparatus is used very carefully and accurately, and can, one hopes, see the high standards set in such a clinic. She can also see how younger children are carefully brought to the point where they can cope with an audiogram, and how the whole situation can be kept as a pleasant experience for the child so that, if he needs to return, his apprehension is decreased and he may even look forward to 'clinic days'.

Secondly, the trainee should spend as long a period as possible with a senior technician in physiological measurement who enjoys working with children. At this stage, the trainee should receive concentrated instruction in air and bone conduction and the techniques of masking. She may, in fact, only be required to use air conduction measurements, but, nevertheless, she should understand the potential of the machine she is going to use, and should realize when bone conduction and masking are going to be necessary even if she does not do them herself. However, sometimes the nurse or technicians are attached to a community health clinic which acts as a second screen before the child is sent on to hospital. In these cases, she must be able to use bone conduction and masking accurately.

Thirdly, the trainee should be thoroughly well aware of other work undertaken by audiological technicians in hospitals. The most important part of this is the use of the *impedance bridge*. With the introduction of machines which make tympanometry measurements so very simple, it seems almost certain that such tympanometers will soon be added to audiometers for use in school screening. In this way, many children with 'glue ear', who are probably missed by audiometry alone, could be picked out, but this is discussed further in Chapter 15.

The pure tone audiometer is a simple machine to use with sufficient practice, but, after the trainee has watched the expert for a reasonable period, she requires a long stint of practice under the supervision of her trainer, followed by a period in which she is working alone but has easy access to her trainer when in difficulty. The length of time required for such a training programme is difficult to estimate; in a busy clinic, the practice facilities may be great and expertise soon acquired. (On the other hand, the experienced technician may be too busy to give much instruction.) In a slack clinic, the trainee may have to practise on the other personnel in the clinic who are able and willing! I think the best advice is to ask the trusted senior technician when he or she feels the trainee has reached a reasonable level of competence, and, if possible, for the doctor in charge of the unit to watch her at work. Before she leaves, she should also be given some insight into the work done with hearing aids; for example, she should be familiar with the appearance of the commonest aids, able to change batteries, aware of how moulds are made and able to insert and take them out, so that she knows when a patient should be referred for new

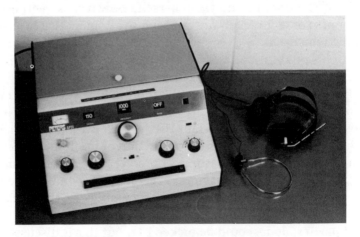

Figure 21   The pure tone audiometer

moulds. She should know the causes of 'whistling' so that she does *not* tell mothers that 'his hearing aid has gone wrong'.

We must now come to a brief description of the machine we have mentioned so many times, the pure tone audiometer. With a skilled operator, this machine can be used on a child with a mental age of around or just over 3 years. The use of the machine depends upon the conditioning process which has been described in detail already (page 84), that is, the child responds to an auditory stimulus by performing a simple motor task. However, the pure tone audiometer has headphones so that the sound may be played into each ear separately. It is sometimes found that a child who has been happy with the conditioning process when using voice, free field audiometer or drum, objects strongly to the use of headphones. On the other hand, if the child has a severe hearing loss and has been receiving auditory training with a

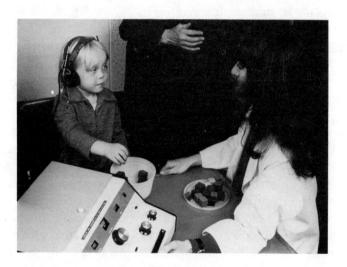

Figure 22   A 3-year old competently doing an audiogram
using a pure tone audiometer

speech trainer under the care of a teacher of the deaf at home, then he is very well acquainted with the headset and this produces no problems. If he is frightened of the earphones, various ploys must be used to dispel his apprehension. His parents and siblings are, again, brought into 'the game' and use the headset in turn; or one earpiece, which is often detachable on a lead from the remainder of the headset, may be put up to the child's ear so that he can hear a succession of tones at different frequencies. In fact, it is sometimes necessary to do the first audiogram by the trainer or the mother holding the earpieces to each ear in turn.

When the child has accepted the earphones, the examiner starts with an appropriate sound at an appropriate frequency in one ear. What do we mean by 'appropriate'? If we have already discovered through distraction tests, preliminary conditioning tests and taking a good history, that we are dealing with a very deaf child, then it may be necessary to start with a maximum sound, which is usually 120 dB, at a low frequency. (Very deaf children, you will remember, often have an island of hearing left in the low frequencies. There are practically *no* children who lack *any* hearing at all.) In such cases, 120 dB at 500 Hz seems a good place to begin. In children where a small conductive loss is suspected, 60 dB at 1 kHz would be a more suitable starting place. In some centres, the child is conditioned with an oscillator before even commencing the loud pure tones.

Once a suitable starting point has been determined, and for most children it is in the middle ranges as suggested above, the technique returns to the familiar performance of carrying out a simple motor task when the child hears the auditory stimulus. As before, he is helped at first, either by examiner or family, until his reliability is established. It is advisable for the examiner to start with a sound which he suspects is well above the child's threshold. In this way, he really conditions to the auditory stimulus and does not confuse the child who then chooses some other stimulus to respond to. (This has already been described in detail in Chapter 9 and the reader will remember how easy it is for the child to respond to some unconscious action on the part of the examiner, such as looking up at the child every time he produces a pure tone in completely regular sequence.) When the child has indicated that he can respond without help, the examiner goes down in 10 dB steps until he obtains no further responses from the child. At this point, he goes up in 5 dB steps until he regains the response. The result is checked and two out of three positive results are acceptable as a result to be marked on the graph.

The examiner then repeats the same examination at 250 Hz, 500 Hz, 1 kHz, 2 kHz and 4 kHz, in each ear in turn. Most audiometers also give pure tones at 125 Hz, 3 kHz, 6 kHz and 8 kHz. This is very useful for some children with specific hearing losses, such as in a child with a very severe loss but residual hearing in the low frequencies, and it is helpful to know the amount of hearing left at 125 Hz. On the other hand, in a child with a high-frequency loss, it is useful to know whether there is reasonable hearing left at 3 kHz and also to know the extent to which the hearing drops at 6 kHz and 8 kHz.

When a very young child does his first audiogram, he will not, of course, have the patience or degree of concentration necessary to give results at all the standard levels. The examiner must pick out those levels which will be most useful to him and attempt these first. When the child shows signs of boredom or impatience, the test should be stopped, the child praised and/or rewarded for his efforts, and more should be attempted at the next test in 3 or 4 months time.

This type of test gives the result of air conduction hearing, that is, the sound travels through the air from the machine, through the middle ear to the inner ear. If there is a hearing loss, this test does not indicate where the lesion lies, whether in the middle ear or the inner ear (cochlea) and/or

8th nerve. As a rule, the smaller hearing loss, worse in the low frequencies, is usually of conductive origin, with the problem lying in the middle ear. The more severe loss, tending to be either flat across all frequencies or worse in the high frequencies, is usually of sensorineural origin. However, it is essential to prove the type of loss and, in order to do this, one must measure bone conduction.

When this is done, the sound is passed straight through the bone to the inner ear, bypassing the middle ear, by placing the vibrator attached to the pure tone audiometer on the mastoid process. As bone is such an excellent conductor of sound, both cochlea respond to the vibrator, on whichever side it is placed and the result obtained simply shows the performance of the better ear. Many people fail to understand that it is quite pointless to measure bone conduction on each side separately *unless* the other ear is 'masked'.

Masking means playing a noise into the ear not under test so that it does not hear the pure tones being played into the ear being tested. The sound used for masking is usually 'narrow-band' noise, or noise containing a narrow spread of frequencies. The volume of noise used must be sufficient to eliminate the possibility of this ear producing a response to the sound being played into the ear being tested. The narrow-band masking noise may be started at around 30 dB and a result obtained for the ear under test. The masking noise is then increased by 10 dB and the ear tested again. If the same result is obtained, the masking noise is again increased by 10 dB. If the result in the ear under test remains the same for three 10 dB increases in masking noise, this result may be taken as valid for that ear.

If, however, one of the 10 dB increases in masking noise results in the ear under test failing to give the same result, then the new result must be found, and the whole process is started again until the three 10 dB increase steps do not affect the response of the tested ear.

In this way, the bone conduction may be measured separately in each ear. If there is a difference between the bone conduction and air conduction levels, it is obvious that there is something preventing adequate conduction of sound through all the structures of the middle ear to the inner ear; for instance, in 'glue ear', there is a typical small gap between the bone conduction, which gives normal results, and the air conduction, which may show low-frequency losses of anything from 30 dB to 50 or 60 dB.

In sensorineural hearing loss, where, as we have said, the lesion lies beyond the middle ear, there is no reason for any difference between bone and air conduction. In fact, on the audiogram, the two normally show close correlation.

It should be remembered, however, that children with a sensorineural hearing loss may also have middle-ear problems, so that a child with a sensorineural loss may show an air–bone gap on his audiogram. Further tests and clinical examination would verify that the child indeed had 'a mixed loss'. In such a case, it may be possible to increase the hearing levels significantly by dealing with the conductive element.

Before leaving the question of masking, one other important use should be mentioned. This is where one ear hears very much better than the other. If there is a 30–40 dB gap between the two ears when air conduction is measured, it is possible that the result in the worse ear is, in fact, improved by the responses coming over from the good ear. In such cases, it is often noticed that the graph given by the bad ear is a 'shadow' of that given by the good ear. A true result for the bad ear can only be obtained by masking the good ear with the method described for bone conduction. A good example of this is often seen in children who have suffered a profound unilateral hearing loss following measles or mumps. A shadow curve with a 50–60 dB difference is always very suspicious and calls for careful masking of the good ear.

Chapter 11

CAUSES OF HEARING LOSS: (a) GENETIC CAUSES

The causes of hearing loss may be conveniently grouped as shown in Table 2 overleaf. It should certainly help the reader not to omit any important cause from conception, through pregnancy, and perinatally until the child is at the age when he is most liable to the common infections. Each of these areas is dealt with briefly below.

GENETIC CAUSES

As will be seen, these can be divided into those cases caused by either dominant genes, recessive genes, or X-linked genes. In each case there is an important subdivision. The child may have a hearing loss caused by one of the three types of gene, but may be normal in every other respect. This is what Fraser[1] calls clinically undifferentiated hearing loss. Thus, we may have autosomal recessive, autosomal dominant or X-linked clinically undifferentiated hearing loss. On the other hand, the hearing loss may be only one part of a whole spectrum of symptoms and signs that are inherited together, either in a dominant, recessive or X-linked fashion. There are many interesting inherited syndromes in which deafness plays a part and which are briefly mentioned below.

Table 2 Causes of hearing loss

Genetic	Causes in pregnancy	Causes around birth	Causes after birth
(1) Autosomal recessive types	(1) Infections, e.g. rubella mumps Cytomegalovirus toxoplasmosis syphilis	(1) Prematurity	(1) Meningitis
(2) Autosomal dominant types		(2) Low birthweight	(2) Other infections, e.g. measles mumps
(3) X-linked recessive types	(2) Drugs (Streptomycin etc.)	(3) Anoxia from any cause	
In all cases, this hearing loss may be either		(4) Raised serum bilirubin in neonatal period	(3) Acquired conductive loss from URTI
(a) Clinically undifferentiated, or			(4) Trauma and noise
(b) Part of a syndrome, e.g. Pendred's syndrome (R) Usher's syndrome (R) Abnormal ECG syndrome (R) (Jervell–Lange–Neilsen) Waardenburg's syndrome (D) Hunter's syndrome (X)			

D = Dominant
R = Recessive
X = Sex-linked

Clinically undifferentiated autosomal recessive hearing loss

This is the commonest type of hearing loss seen in children. Fraser discovered an incidence of 25% in the school study done in the British Isles.

In some cases, where no apparent cause can be found for the hearing loss, it is thought that this may be due to mutation of a gene.

Clinically undifferentiated autosomal recessive hearing loss has certain recognizable features. First of all, there is the situation where two 'normal' parents produce more than one deaf child. A similar situation is where consanguineous parents, both hearing normally, produce a deaf child. Secondly, this is usually a very severe form of sensorineural deafness, tending to be worse in the high than the low frequencies. Hence, we often see what is colloquially called 'a left-hand corner audiogram' (Figure 23). This clearly

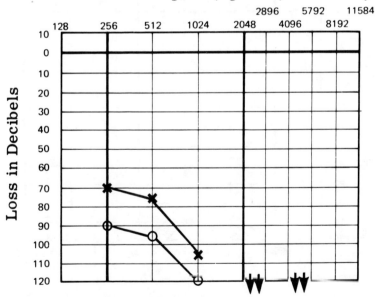

Figure 23   Clinically undifferentiated autosomal recessive hearing loss: typical audiogram; ○ right ear. × left ear

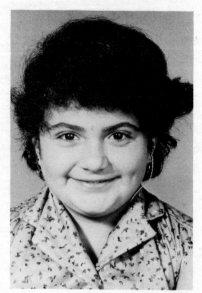

Fig 24a

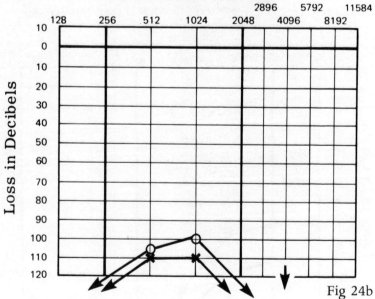

Fig 24b

Figure 24 (a) A 5-year-old girl with profound autosomal recessive hearing loss whose parents are first cousins with normal hearing. (b) Her audiogram. No bone conduction recorded; ○ right ear. × left ear

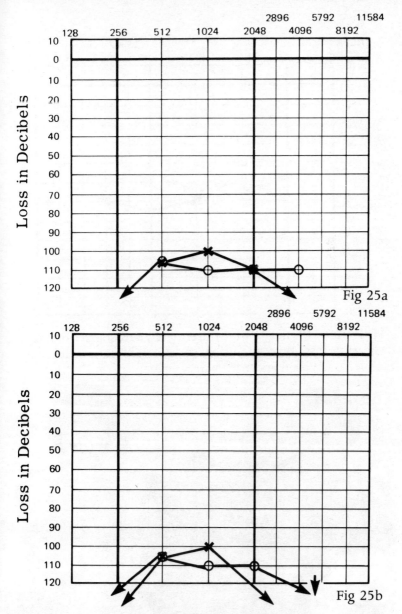

Figure 25 Audiograms of two siblings with normally hearing parents and one older normally hearing brother. Both have autosomal recessive hearing loss. No bone conduction recorded. (a) C. aged 5 years. (b) E. aged 3 years; ◯ right ear. × left ear

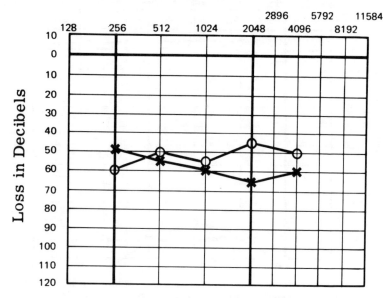

Figure 26   Clinically undifferentiated autosomal dominant hearing loss: typical audiogram; ○ right ear; × left ear

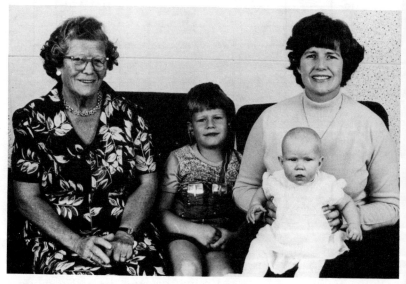

Figure 27   Three generations showing an autosomal dominant hearing loss. Tests on the baby are not yet complete, but she probably has normal hearing

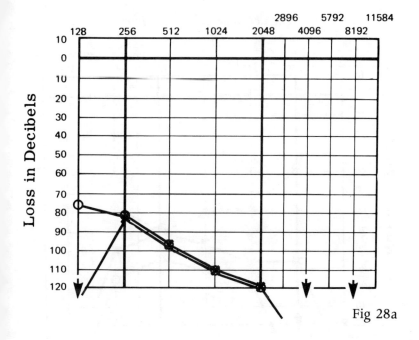

Fig 28a

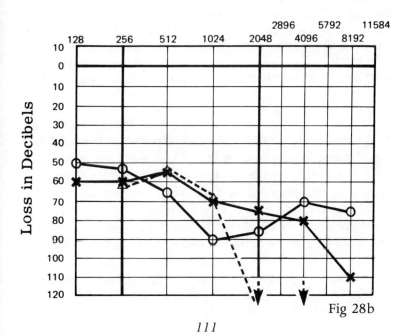

Fig 28b

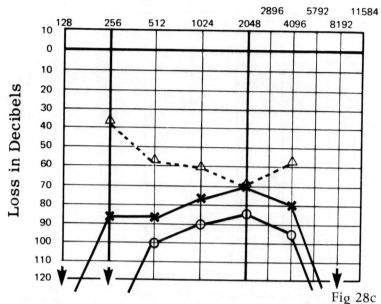

Fig 28c

Figure 28   The audiograms of the family shown in Figure 27.
(a) S, aged 7 years; note that his audiogram is *not* typical of the
dominant-type hearing loss – he hears less than any other
member of his family; No bone conduction is recorded. (b)
The mother of patient S: Δ --- unmasked bone conduction.
(c) The maternal grandmother of patient S: Δ --- unmasked
bone conduction; ◯ right ear; ✕ left ear

shows that the island of hearing remaining in the low
frequencies often enables such children to hear low-flying
aircraft and loud traffic noise, which, as I have previously
said, contain a high proportion of low-frequency sounds. It
should be remembered that it is very rare indeed to find a
child without *any* measurable hearing.

By contrast, *clinically undifferentiated autosomal dominant
hearing loss* tends to be rather less severe than the recessive
variety. In fact, although in many cases it can be seen in
grandparents, great aunts or uncles, etc., it may sometimes
appear to 'miss' a generation. If the investigator is lucky

enough to be able to test some of the 'missed' generation, he may well find one or two cases where the loss has been so small that it has caused no special educational or social problems but, nevertheless, a small loss can be demonstrated audiometrically. Of course, this happened particularly before the days of routine tests and the patient's family did not consider it a handicap or seek advice. Another thing that may be found in such an investigation is a unilateral hearing loss. In addition to the fact that the dominant type of hearing loss is often less severe than the recessive type, it also tends to be equally severe across the frequencies. This generally means that the child has a better chance of acquiring reasonable speech as he tends to hear many more consonants than the unfortunate child with a 'left-hand corner audiogram'.

In the majority of cases of autosomal dominant loss, the loss *can* be found in each generation as far as the family's knowledge extends. Thus we have parents, grandparents, aunts, uncles and cousins, etc. who can be traced.

Clinically undifferentiated autosomal dominant cases accounted for 11.6% of the children studied in the British Isles by Fraser[1].

The last type of clinically undifferentiated hearing loss, *X-linked*, is extremely rare. Fraser[1] recounts two interesting families only, out of his striking survey of the literature of the last century. (There appears to have been great interest in deafness in families at that time and a considerable documentation is available.) The first tells of a family in Berlin in 1836, where an investigator named Kramer, who was one of the first really scientific investigators, appears to have been fascinated by a family of six sons and five daughters. Both parents had normal hearing and were not aware of any other deaf relatives, but their six sons were all 'deaf-mutes' while their five daughters were entirely normal. The other family was described in 1898 and consisted of two deaf brothers with a deaf uncle and a deaf nephew.

Since this time many families have been recorded where the sons had a hearing loss, whereas their sisters were normal. There have been a very few cases where such a situation has been traced in more than one generation. Generally, in these cases the hearing loss seems to produce a relatively flat audiogram, and *not* the type worse in the high frequencies as seen in the autosomal recessive group.

Autosomal recessive syndromes

Pendred's syndrome

This was first described by Dr Vaughan Pendred, in the *Lancet* in 1896. He was a country general practitioner, but described himself in the *Lancet* as 'Late House Surgeon to Guy's Hospital'.

The syndrome is inherited in recessive fashion and has well-defined clinical features, easily remembered when one thinks of it as 'Pendred's syndrome' or 'deafness with goitre'. The enlargement of the thyroid is due to its inability to change the inorganic iodide normally ingested in the diet, to an acceptable organic form which can be used to form thyroxine, because of the absence of the required enzyme. In fact, in order to try and overcome this deficiency the thyroid becomes very enlarged and manages, normally, to keep the patient in a euthyroid state. The test, which is absolutely diagnostic for this condition is the perchlorate test (Table 3).

The type of deafness present is usually that already described under autosomal recessive hearing loss, but this is not always the case. (The writer looks after a proven case of Pendred's syndrome where a considerable part of the hearing loss was found to be due to 'glue ear'. After treatment of this, the remaining loss was really very mild, but still tended to show a loss worse in the low frequencies and, of course, a sensorineural low-frequency hearing loss.)

Causes of hearing loss

Pendred's syndrome must not be confused with the hearing loss that is often found in children with untreated hypothyroidism. Lack of thyroid *in utero* appears to affect the developing cochlea.

Table 3   Principle of perchlorate test: diagnostic of Pendred's syndrome

---

(1)   Perchlorate ions (ClO_4^-) are capable of discharging inorganic iodide from thyroid gland.
(2)   In the normal thyroid gland, the inorganic iodide is quickly transformed to the organic form and *very little* inorganic form is left in the gland.

The test
(1)   Give the patient a dose of radioactive inorganic iodide; take a Geiger count.
(2)   Give the patient a dose of potassium perchlorate ($KClO_4$).
(3)   The normal gland will have *used* the radioactive iodide and converted it to an organic form; but the iodine remains *in* the gland, simply in another form.
(4)   In Pendred's disease the gland cannot use the inorganic iodide, therefore the perchlorate discharges it *away* from the gland.
(5)   Take another Geiger count, over the gland; in the normal gland the *count remains the same*, as the radioiodine remains *in* the gland, simply in another form.

In Pendred's disease the radioactive iodide has been 'discharged from the gland' as it has stayed in *inorganic form*. Therefore the Geiger count *over the gland* falls as the radioactive iodide has been sent off to other parts of the body by the potassium perchlorate.

Usher's syndrome

Usher's syndrome was first described rather earlier than Pendred's syndrome. In fact it was the discovery of the ophthalmoscope that indirectly led to the discovery of this syndrome consisting of an association between deafness and retinitis pigmentosa. In 1861, a worker by the name of Liebreich surveyed the number of cases in which retinitis pigmentosa occurred in the deaf, although Usher in 1914 finally gave his name to the condition, and several other workers made similar surveys at times varying from 1907 until the present time[1].

The full picture of Usher's syndrome is not commonly seen in young patients, because although the deafness is of very early onset and is probably diagnosed at the same time as clinically undifferentiated autosomal recessive deafness, the symptoms in the eyes do not usually commence until late childhood or in adult life. It is possible, of course, that if electrodiagnostic tests were carried out on the eyes of all deaf children then the signs would be found in infancy, thus long preceding the onset of ordinary clinical signs and symptoms. As it is, the disease is sometimes found, almost accidentally, when a middle-aged deaf person has his eyes tested, and the typical peripheral lesions are found on ophthalmoscopic examination. Clinically, the patient may develop tunnel vision or night blindness as first symptoms, and cataracts may form in later life. However, the prognosis for vision varies very widely. Retinal changes may remain minimal and stationary and cataracts may not form. On the other hand retinal changes may advance, causing very serious degeneration, and if cataracts also play a part, then the patient may become blind.

The hearing loss tends to be of the same 'shape' as that found in other cases of autosomal recessive deafness, that is, usually worse in the high frequencies, but the degree varies in different individuals. It should be noted, however, that post-mortem findings sometimes show that in addition to widespread degeneration in the organ of Corti there are also changes in the vestibular apparatus. Thus, vestibular disturbance is much more common in Usher's syndrome than in any other form of inherited deafness. This is particularly unfortunate when a patient who is already deaf, and whose sight is deteriorating, shows ataxia due to vestibular involvement.

Obviously it is very important that the vision of young deaf children is tested regularly; this can be appreciated from several different angles, as well as from the diagnostic view of Usher's disease. The very young deaf baby is usually intensely 'visual' in his behaviour, seeking to increase his experience of the world by this means as one of the other sensory inputs is so limited for him. As he reaches the stage of auditory training, lip-reading forms a vital part of his education from an immensely early age. In addition, if he is taught an alternative means of communication (see Chapter 14) he needs optimal vision to develop this to his best advantage.

Laurence–Moon–Bardet–Biedl syndrome

This comparatively unusual syndrome is mentioned because most textbooks omit deafness when describing it. It is a condition in which pituitary dystrophy, retinitis pigmentosa and polydactyly are associated; mental handicap may, or may not, be present.

The author, however, has under her care three cases in which deafness is present. In one case, which has been followed for several years, deafness did not occur until the child was around 6 years of age, although he was already attending a school for the blind. In the second case, too, it appears that deafness has definitely been appearing with age. Both these cases are now using hearing aids.

The development of hearing

Abnormal ECG syndrome (*Jervell and Lange-Neilsen syndrome*)

While Pendred's syndrome is said to account for about 5% of severe hearing loss in children and Usher's syndrome 1.2% (adults around 4%), abnormal ECG syndrome is really very rare, accounting for only about 0.7% of all cases in Fraser's study in the British Isles.

However, this is such an intriguing and interesting condition that it deserves a brief mention. Here a hearing loss of the autosomal recessive type is associated with typical changes in the electrocardiogram. In fact it seems a distinct possibility that some infants with this condition die before their hearing loss has been discovered.

The clinical symptoms are those of unexplained 'fainting' attacks, and in fact it was not until 1957 that when Jervell and Lange-Nielsen described a family containing four affected children, attention moved from possible neurological to possible cardiac causes. In fact the EEGs of such children are entirely normal while the ECGs show typical changes. Unfortunately, one of the fainting attacks finally proves fatal, usually before adolescence, although females tend to survive rather longer than males.

The Germans, who as we have seen seem to have written assiduously about deafness in children, during the last century recorded several cases of sudden death which were probably examples of this condition. The most dramatic was that of a little girl who was being rebuked, in public, for a very minor piece of misbehaviour, in a Leipzig school for the deaf around 1856. She promptly collapsed and died. In addition, she was found to have had two sisters who died very suddenly, one after a fright and the other after a fit of temper[1].

In fact it is now realized that the 'faints' are precipitated by exercise, by emotion and also by quinidine. The only treatment that appears to have some normalizing effect on the ECG is digitalis, which is used as long-term therapy when this condition has been diagnosed before it becomes fatal.

It also seems very possible that this condition is responsible for a small number of 'undiagnosed' cot deaths.

The typical finding in the ECG is a lengthening of the QT interval, which is due to an increase in length of the ST portion and the T wave. The QRS section appears normal. Fright, etc., produces other changes in the T wave, which may become inverted and biphasic. Sometimes the biphasic T wave becomes almost confluent with the P wave following it.

There are no other findings on clinical examination of the heart, and some post-mortem findings have reported abnormalities of the conductive system in the heart, that is abnormalities of the Purkinje fibres and of the sinus node, which are responsible for the passage of normal electrical impulses through the heart.

Pathological changes found in the ear in recessive conditions

Knowledge about this is extremely limited. As has already been mentioned, in Usher's syndrome widespread degeneration of the cells in the organ of Corti has been found, together with degeneration of the vestibular apparatus cells. Very little seems to be known about the changes in Pendred's disease, although one post-mortem in 1968 showed an abnormality of the bony structure of the labyrinth, which seemed a very surprising finding. In fact this type of abnormality has been shown to be quite clearly associated with autosomal dominant hearing loss. In the abnormal ECG syndrome the organ of Corti has been found to be severely affected and degenerated, with retraction of the tectorial membrane. Abnormalities of both the cochlear and vestibular areas of the membranous labyrinth were found, with abnormal material lying within the blood vessels, and on the spiral prominence containing the very important spiral ganglion. The same abnormal material was found in such quantities in the horizontal semicircular canal that it was unrecognizable. In this respect, the degenerative condition resembled that found in Usher's disease.

In clinically undifferentiated autosomal recessive deafness the degeneration has usually been found to be limited to the cochlea and the saccule, with haemorrhages and thromboses in the important tiny vessels that supply the 8th nerve endings.

The most interesting area of discussion lies, however, in the question of *when* this degeneration takes place and *how* it is that deafness is associated with such disparate conditions in the varying syndromes. Evidence from animals suggests that in many hereditary forms of deafness, the degeneration is *not* present at birth, but occurs very quickly after it. There is a very important analogy here with phenylketonuria. If degeneration is not present at birth eventually it should be possible to prevent its commencement. Obviously there is a wide field for research here.

If the above theory is correct it provides an explanation for the occasional cases of autosomal recessive hearing loss that regress. While there is no doubt at all that almost every case should be diagnosed before the first birthday, as we have already stressed, there are occasional cases which do not appear until the second or, very occasionally, even the third year of life. This is another reason why hearing tests should be made regularly at the recommended intervals, even when the initial examination, done correctly, has yielded perfect results in a normal baby.

Autosomal dominant syndromes

These mainly consist of what are known as the *auditory-pigmentary syndromes*, an almost self-explanatory title. The most important one (and we shall limit ourselves to describing this) is *Waardenburg's syndrome*. In 1951 he described the various signs and symptoms, showing how they occurred together, forming a well-marked syndrome, inherited in a dominant fashion.

The reader has probably seen a case of this syndrome, which in its entirety is very striking, but may not have realized its significance. In the 'total' syndrome the following components are seen:

(1) A white forelock. This may be very marked or the examiner may have to hunt to find a few white hairs hidden under the normally coloured front hair. In some cases the whole of the hair is very fair, or lacking in pigment. There is a tendency for all these patients to develop grey hair at an unusually early age and to have hair of poor quality.

(2) Heterochromia, or different-coloured eyes. This may be total, such as blue with green, blue with brown, etc., or segments of the iris may be of a different colour. Sometimes both eyes are of a very pale blue colour, again showing a lack of pigment. Hypopigmentation of the fundus is also sometimes present and, occasionally, the abnormalities of the eyes lead to glaucoma in young patients.

(3) 'Dystopia canthi medialis lateroversa' or lateral displacement of the medial canthi of the eyes. This simply means that if one looks straight into the patient's eyes, there is very little sclera visible between the medial canthus of the eye and the pupil. The examiner's first impression of the patient may be that his eyes are not normal and that he has an unusually broad and prominent root to the nose. More careful observation will then show this to be due to dystopia of the medial canthi. (The lucky examiner can then see the heterochromia, although this is not always present.) The eyebrows may also be confluent.

(4) Two types of hearing loss may be present, this having been well demonstrated by Fisch in 1959. He showed that

the first group had the pigmentary anomalies associated with a very severe hearing loss, that is the type normally associated with recessive type loss, while the second group retained much more hearing, with no deterioration in the higher frequencies. In other words the second group showed the usual dominant type of loss. An extraordinary finding was that the two ears in one individual might show the two types of hearing loss.

(5) Other findings in this syndrome include other pigmentary anomalies, or areas of hypopigmentation of the skin, but oddly enough there may also be areas of hyperpigmentation, as in freckles and nevi. The skin may therefore be very patchy and the term 'piebald' can sometimes be aptly ascribed to it.

It is rare to find all the symptoms and signs described in any one individual. Various permutations and combinations seem to occur, but the presence of dystopia with deafness is considered to be the essential diagnostic element.

Pathological findings appear to be limited to degeneration of the cells of the organ of Corti, without any bony or vestibular abnormalities. However, the vascular supply is affected, as is the spiral ganglion which also shows degeneration.

Other autosomal dominant syndromes

There are a few other syndromes, inherited in this way, which the reader may also come across. The first is *Alport's syndrome* in which nephritis is associated with sensorineural hearing loss. There is also an interesting syndrome in which renal tubular acidosis in children is associated with sensorineural hearing loss. It is thought to be inherited as a recessive trait[2]. The deafness usually becomes worse as the child becomes older, so it is often insignificant, before adolescence. The writer has a patient who has, in fact, had a successful kidney transplant. He has a moderate, flat, sensorineural hearing loss which would be easily treatable by two postaural hearing aids. These are now so small and inconspicuous that by judicious arrangement of the hair – even in adolescent boys – they are practically invisible (in girls, of course, they are very easily completely hidden). Unhappily he is very unwilling to attempt to use these aids, which would certainly make life easier for him. His family, feeling he is a very 'special' boy, in view of his medical history, are very indulgent to him and give me no support in my persuasive efforts. I recount this episode to show the reader that when a hearing aid is prescribed a family often puts up immediate barriers with a multitude of rationalizations to show why their child should not use an aid. One understands only too well the feelings of parents whose handsome, beautiful baby has to wear two body-worn aids, yet one finds that the same feelings quite often even extend to the use of the modern, tiny postaural aids. More will be said about this in Chapter 18 but in the meantime I continue to persuade this particular family that aids would not only make life much easier for their child as he leaves school, and starts a job, but would make life much more interesting and more fun, instead of continuing his perpetual struggle to hear an instruction, a question or a joke.

Malformations of the branchial arches, occurring *in utero*, may sometimes be inherited in a dominant manner. The best known of these is the *Treacher–Collins syndrome* or mandibulofacial dysostosis. This includes abnormalities of the outer and middle ears, and sometimes also of the inner ear. The eyes tend to show an anti-mongoloid slant, with colobomas of the lower eyelids. As the name implies there is marked hypoplasia both of the malar bone and the mandible. There may also be macrostomia, with a high palate and malformed teeth, and blind fistulae occurring in the area between the angles of the mouth and the ears. As with the auditory–pigmentary syndromes not all the features need be present together, but various permutations and combinations may be seen, as well as varying degrees of severity.

In my clinic we look after one boy who has the syndrome in a very severe form. Tomograms have shown him to have grossly disorganized middle ears, with some abnormality of the inner ears. He has no external ears or external auditory canals, but some accessory auricles. Surgery, which was done before he came to the care of our clinic, attempted to improve the shape of his face by inserting plastic material in the area of the underdeveloped malar bones. This has, in fact, been very unsuccessful and only the scars remain. The tomograms, of course, indicate that there is no point in attempting further surgery, in view of the very poor condition of the middle ear. In addition to his gross communication problem he is also mentally handicapped. However, we have been able to show that his inner ear, although abnormal in appearance, must contain normal hearing elements, as we have taught him to respond to the bone conductor on the audiometer, in fact we have shown him to have hearing within normal limits when measured by this method. We are, therefore, treating him with a bone conduction hearing aid, that is an aid where the mould or earpiece is replaced by a vibrator anchored to the mastoid process by means of a headband. He will, of course, never speak or comprehend speech, particularly as this treatment was not started until we got to know him at about the age of 8 years. However, we aim to give him some pleasure and stimulation through sound, and possibly to provide him with a warning system. We may enable him to comprehend the word 'No' by a mixture of sound, facial expression and gesture, which can be very useful (see Chapter 16).

Deafness is also occasionally associated with the *Pierre Robin syndrome*, another branchial arch anomaly. In this case, a cleft palate is associated with characteristic under-development of the mandible. This is almost certainly inherited in a dominant fashion, although in common with all the other dominant syndromes described, it varies very much in severity and quite often malformation of the mandible is present with a normal palate. Fortunately, as the child grows older the mandible tends to grow too, so that in adult life the person may appear completely normal.

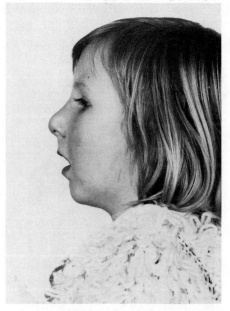

Figure 29 Child with Pierre Robin syndrome

Many other combinations of symptoms and signs, associated with hearing loss and obviously inherited in a dominant fashion, have been reported by individual workers. One of the most interesting families (Figure 30) attending my clinic at the moment shows a combination of multiple epiphyseal dysplasia tarda with osteochondromatosis and sensorineural hearing loss. The mother of my young patient has recently had a hip replacement operation for severe and disabling 'osteoarthritis' at a very young age. (NB: I am here using the term 'osteoarthritis' *only* as it is used by the family.) She also has a typical dominant-type hearing loss. Her only child, a girl of 3, was referred to me because of a possible mild hearing loss. This appears to be present in a very mild form, not yet requiring amplification, but her mother's hearing loss was also insignificant until adolescence. There is a very well-marked family history of 'osteoarthritis' associated with sensorineural hearing loss. The mode of inheritance is typically dominant and the onset of hearing loss has tended to be in adolescence or later. I am awaiting further family enquiries before drawing up as complete a family tree as possible.

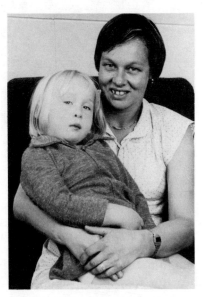

Figure 30   Two members of the family (see text) showing an association between 'osteoarthritis' and deafness inherited in dominant fashion

Lastly, we must mention *otosclerosis* which is also inherited in a dominant manner. I have left this until last, as the deafness here is wholly conductive in type, while all the other conditions mentioned above produce either sensorineural deafness or, in the case of the branchial arch conditions, usually a mixture of sensorineural and conductive deafness, although many cases in this category may be limited to conductive deafness only. (Such cases include the group where there is asymmetry or atresia of the external ear, associated with earpits, accessory auricles and sinuses between the ear and the mouth and in the neck, in other words, *deafness–earpits syndrome*). In addition, otosclerosis has been left to this stage because of its time of onset. It is not usually seen in children, but appears in adolescence or later life. The name 'otosclerosis' means a hardening of the bone, but as Ballantyne[3] points out this is very misleading. The petrous portion of the temporal bone (so named after Peter or 'The Rock') is, in fact, one of the hardest areas of bone in the body. Otosclerosis actually consists of a condition in which the normal hard bone is replaced by spongy bone of an immature type, usually beginning in the region of the promontory of the middle ear. It will be remembered from Chapter 4 that the oval window is placed above the posterior end of the promontory and the condition spreads slowly to involve the margins of the oval window. But, again, remembering the close relationship between the stapes and the oval window, the disease process can easily spread to involve the highly important footplate of the stapes, and it finally causes the footplate to become fixed. This simply means that the whole process of conduction of sound as described in Chapter 4 is severely interrupted and the patient becomes more and more deaf. The cochlea is only very rarely involved, so this is a conductive type of deafness; on the audiogram the air conduction shows the hearing loss while the bone conduction remains normal, except for a little 'notch' around 2 kHz (2000 Hz) which is known as Carhart's notch and is diagnostic of stapedial fixation.

As has already been stated, symptoms are first noticed in the late 'teens or in the twenties, and women seem to be affected twice as often as men, particularly as it seems to be aggravated by childbirth.

Fortunately, surgical treatment of the condition (stapedectomy) is very effective, and when a case is suspected the patient should be sent at once for surgical opinion.

Pathological findings in autosomal dominant hearing loss

It must be stressed that, although we have already discussed changes found in both recessive and dominant types of hearing loss, the total body of knowledge is really very small indeed.

In general it can probably be said that while recessive conditions show pathological changes limited to the cochlea and the organ of Corti, in particular, the dominant conditions more often involve the whole of the inner ear. However, there are so many exceptions to this generalization that perhaps one should simply say that here is another area where much more work needs to be done.

X-linked syndromes

We have already seen that clinically undifferentiated X-linked hearing loss is rare. But the best known syndrome involving hearing loss, and inherited in X-linked fashion, is one of the mucopolysaccharides, *Hunter's syndrome*. In this condition there is dwarfism, associated with coarsening of the facial features, which has led to the use of the term 'gargoylism'. Deafness is a common finding in boys with Hunter's syndrome. The degree of mental handicap seems to vary enormously and the writer looks after several cases, with varying degrees of intelligence. One little 7-year-old boy is of completely normal intelligence, with a most pleasant and attractive personality, who finds no problem at all in using postaural hearing aids to good effect. However, it should be remembered that these children tend to deteriorate as more abnormal material, resulting from abnormal metabolism of the high molecular carbohydrates, is laid down in cells all over the body. My cases also include several children with profound mental handicap.

The other forms of mucopolysaccharidosis, of which there are many, are probably inherited in a recessive fashion, and there is no doubt that deafness is sometimes found in these syndromes, although not as commonly as in Hunter's syndrome. The author looks after one little girl with *Hurler's syndrome* who has a moderate, flat-shaped hearing loss. This was, in fact, first noticed by the clinical psychologist who was assessing her abilities. She was quickly referred to my clinic and just as she was becoming accustomed to the use of two postaural aids, she tragically had an acute onset of blindness. This was too acute to be attributed to corneal clouding, which is a feature of Hurler's disease, but was thought to be due to an acute episode in the brain, probably associated with one of the cystic areas that are associated with large balloon cells distended with the abnormal storage material.

Another patient well known to my clinic has *Sanfilippo syndrome*. She is very severely retarded, and is degenerating, and has a moderate hearing loss.

Children with these syndromes probably have a mixture of conductive and sensorineural hearing loss, due to the presence of abnormal material throughout the ear. If the conductive element is treated by myringotomy, with clearing of the contents of the middle ear and insertion of grommets, although there may be a very temporary improvement recurrence is often found, and in that case amplification should be used rather than more surgery. However, there is no reason why such children should not also get ordinary glue ear, in which case surgical treatment may be very helpful.

References

1. Fraser, G.R. (1976). *The Causes of Profound Deafness in Childhood*. (London: Baillière Tindall)

2. Dunger, D.B., Brenton, D.P. and Cain, A.R. (1980). Renal tubular acidosis and nerve deafness. *Arch. Dis. Child.*, **55**, 221

3. Ballantyne, J. (1978). *Deafness.* (Edinburgh: Churchill Livingstone)

Chapter 12

CAUSES OF HEARING LOSS: (b) OTHER CAUSES

Having discussed the inherited forms of hearing loss we must pass on to the further groups, particularly those causes arising from infections in pregnancy. That is the chief group dealt with in this chapter.

RUBELLA

The tragedy of *rubella* occurring during pregnancy has already been mentioned (page 24), and the particular tragedy is that this is a preventable disease. I must say again here that we have an enormous responsibility in drawing the attention of all the families that we see, wherever and at what ever age we see them (grandchildren, aunts, cousins, etc. may be lurking at home in an 'unimmunized' state) to the absolute necessity of rubella vaccination for girls of 11 years onwards, during the child-bearing period of life. If a girl is unsure as to whether she has already had rubella then she should have a blood test done to ascertain the antibody titre. In any case it is probably a wise move for *all* girls and young women in this category to have this test, as many of those who report a 'definite' history of rubella find that their antibody titre shows that they have insufficient protection and, in fact, need a vaccination.

Congenital rubella results from the attack of the virus on

the fetus during the first trimester of pregnancy, and the earlier the attack the worse is the damage inflicted on the fetus. Other problems (see also Chapter 2) include lesions of the eyes, such as cataracts and the typical rubella choroido-retinitis, so that probably the commonest cause of deaf–blind children is the congenital rubella syndrome. Heart lesions are common and the newborn infant shows hepatospleno-megaly and, sometimes, a purpuric rash. Microcephaly is very common, and is accompanied by mental subnormality. At its worst, therefore, the child with a full rubella syndrome presents as a severely mentally handicapped child, with deafness, visual defect of varying degree and a possible heart lesion. It is this tragedy that we must aim to eradicate with all the vigour that was put into the fight against polio. I can personally remember the long queues of children coming to me for protection against polio when the vaccine was first available, but I have noticed no comparable enthusiasm about the rubella programme, and this is due to public ignorance and some medical inertia, which we must combat vigorously.

If the 'rubella child' is lucky he may escape with a hearing loss alone. This tends to happen when the infection has occurred right at the end of the first trimester of pregnancy. The hearing loss has an *occasional* tendency to become worse during the first and second years of life, but very rarely indeed after this (the infant may continue to excrete rubella virus for some months after birth). It is also quite often characterized by being 'saucer-shaped' in type, that is, the worst loss being in the middle frequencies with improved hearing in the lower and higher frequencies. Although usually it is a very severe loss, I have one or two patients with only a moderate loss.

Examination at autopsy in young infants has shown the pathology of the inner ear to be very similar to that found in inherited recessive loss.

CYTOMEGALOVIRUS (CMV)

As mentioned above, other infections in pregnancy must not be forgotten. The *cytomegalovirus* (*CMV*) has been shown recently to damage the developing ears, although the commonest problems are found in the eyes, with accompanying subnormality. I have a small patient, who has eye lesions, mild mental subnormality and a marked hearing loss, due to a CMV infection in pregnancy. She has now gone to a special boarding school (which takes children with a hearing loss and one other handicap, usually but not invariably mild mental retardation) having already spent some time in a normal partially hearing unit. She has been using hearing aids regularly for many years after an initial battle to get her to use them at home as well as at school. At the age of 8 years she has settled well into the boarding school and is able to communicate with speech at around a $2\frac{1}{2}$ to 3 year level. This may well improve when a manual communication system is added to purely oral methods of education.

OTHER CAUSES IN PREGNANCY

The great danger of the CMV virus is the insidious nature of its attack in pregnancy, and this also applies to *toxoplasmosis* which, again, may affect the developing ear of the fetus, while leaving the mother unscathed. Fortunately, toxoplasmosis is a rare cause of hearing loss.

Measles and *mumps* in pregnancy have also been cited as responsible for damage to the fetal cochlea. *Syphilis* was formerly a common cause of deafness, but fortunately is now rare in this country.

Drugs given during pregnancy may be dangerous to the developing ear. Streptomycin and particularly dihydrostreptomycin and allied drugs seem to have the ability to damage the nerve supply of the inner ear. In those cases where thalidomide damaged the ears, the damage was usually of a very 'total' nature, with involvement of the auricle and middle ears as well as destruction of both parts of the inner ear.

In perinatal causes we must start by mentioning the risk of deafness occurring in premature and small-for-dates babies. In these infants the blood vessels supplying the cochlea are immature and the tendency to haemorrhages in the inner ear is increased. In addition to the decreased blood supply to the organ of Corti, any blood extravasated into this area appears to have a toxic and irreversible effect on the cells of the area[1]. Forceps delivery in such infants appears to increase the possibility of haemorrhage.

ANOXIA AS AN INDIRECT CAUSE OF HEARING LOSS

Anoxia occurring before, during or after birth, may be the result of many obstetric hazards. Severe toxaemia of pregnancy, associated with infarction of the placenta, may cause quite a long period of 'chronic' anoxia to the fetus before birth. Difficult fetal positions, such as transverse lie, breech with extended legs, etc. may result in long labours culminating in difficult deliveries, with signs of fetal distress. Fortunately most obstetricians now actively intervene and prevent long periods of anoxia occurring before and during delivery. Emergencies, such as prolapsed cord or placenta praevia, may cause anoxia unless treatment is swiftly available. Respiratory distress syndrome or hyaline membrane disease can also cause serious anoxia after birth unless the infant can be treated very rapidly in a special care unit, where blood gases are monitored efficiently.

Anoxia due to any of the above causes – or any other cause – may result not only in haemorrhage in the inner ear but also in damage to the cochlear nuclei in the brain.

JAUNDICE

Jaundice is a considerable danger in the newborn period.

This may be due to Rh or AB–O incompatibilities, or to excessive physiological jaundice in a small or premature infant. In any case, the products resulting from the breakdown of the red blood cells are too great to be dealt with by the liver and are therefore carried by the blood-stream and deposited in various parts of the body. It would appear that the deafness resulting from these conditions is due to the deposition of these toxic products in the cochlear nuclei of the brain. The other areas usually affected are the basal ganglia, thus resulting in athetoid cerebral palsy, but the other cranial nuclei may also be affected.

The subject is dealt with in more detail in Chapter 16, but it must be stressed here that, because of the selective areas in which the unconjugated bilirubin is laid down, the patient, although athetoid and deaf, may have a considerable degree of intelligence preserved. The problem, however, remains one of extraordinarily difficult communication, so it is extremely important to make every possible effort to assess the patient's intelligence correctly and to give him every possible opportunity of learning. Sign systems are often of immense value and there are now a variety of machines which enable the patient to communicate in spite of what seem almost insuperable difficulties. The Spastics Society has a range of educational establishments which cater specially for children with other problems added to their motor difficulties.

In some cases the hearing loss is not accompanied by gross motor problems but only by 'minor' problems, such as a very marked degree of clumsiness which can be very troublesome in childhood.

The aim, however, of the obstetrician and neonatal paediatrician is to prevent the level of the serum bilirubin reaching a danger level. Certainly 18 mg/100 ml, *and possibly less*[2], is dangerous, and at around this stage especially if the level is rising a total replacement transfusion is usually undertaken to remove the toxic substances from the infant's circulation. After this the child is carefully observed, in case a 'top-up' transfusion is required.

Prophylaxis is also possible now. The danger of incompatibility arises *after* the first pregnancy when the mother has been sensitized by the first infant's cells and produced antibodies against them. If she can be desensitized after the first pregnancy then subsequent infants are much safer. This is now done by giving the mother anti-D immunoglobulin after the first pregnancy (it is, in fact, given in the postpartum period before the mother leaves hospital).

OTHER POSTNATAL CAUSES OF HEARING LOSS

Given that the infant has passed safely through its life *in utero*, through the birth process and the early postnatal period and given that it has not received abnormal genes from its parents, what are the remaining dangers that may cause a hearing loss in childhood? Perhaps first we should mention the question of drugs as many ill infants are only enabled to survive by the use of ototoxic drugs. This often causes paediatricians considerable anxiety and they are extremely careful to monitor the blood levels of the commonly used, and potentially ototoxic drugs, such as gentamicin. Obviously this can pose very difficult questions to those in charge of the sick neonate, who possibly might only survive by the use of relatively heavy doses of drugs known to be dangerous in another area. Similar questions may arise in the treatment of a few cases of meningitis, who prove resistant to the normally used triad of chloramphenicol, penicillin and sulphonamide.

MENINGITIS

Meningitis is the most dangerous source of sensorineural deafness to which the child is likely to succumb in later childhood. We have already said that a general figure of 5% seems, from a survey of the literature, to be about the right estimate of children likely to be left with a very severe sensorineural hearing loss after an attack of meningitis, even without use of ototoxic drugs. However, reports from various parts of the world have, in fact, produced widely differing figures. (For example, a report from China said that 25% of the cases treated in an otolaryngology service were due to meningitis. Obviously this figure cannot be realistically compared with figures from the western world, but nevertheless a survey made in 1962, in Northumberland and Durham, in a group of schoolchildren with hearing loss, came up with the same figure, that is 25% due to meningitis!). In my own clinic, where we see around 400 children in a year, I am at the moment treating nine children with hearing loss following meningitis, or 2.25% of the children referred to a highly specialized clinic.

We have already said that the causative organism, and the progression of the illness, including time of diagnosis, and incidence of complications such as fits, coma etc. does not seem to show any correlation with the subsequent development of hearing loss. In fact one of my small patients, aged 3 years, complained to his mother that he could not hear *before* the diagnosis was made and he was admitted to hospital. It must be added that in his case there was a delay of 3 days before final diagnosis and admission to hospital. In another of my cases, where the meningitis was in the neonatal period, and a wrong diagnosis of craniostenosis was originally made, thus causing a severe delay in treatment with the subsequent onset of fits, apnoea etc., the final degree of hearing loss is the least severe of any of my group of nine cases. It could be said, therefore, that the incidence of hearing loss after meningitis is capricious.

On the whole the hearing loss is profound (see audiograms); all but two of my own nine cases have a profound loss. An interesting point, which requires further research, is that these two patients received steroids during treatment; in one case this was due to the grave severity of the

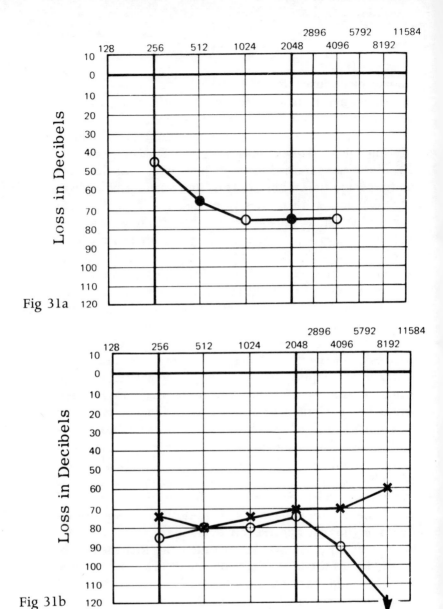

Figure 31 (a) A, aged 14 months with post-meningitic loss, treated with steroids (free field audiometry). ● Stilling plus eye movement; ○ turn plus indications that he heard before the above levels were reached. (b) S, aged 4 years with post-meningitic loss, treated with steroids; no bone conductions recorded; ○ right ear, × left ear

course of the illness, and in the second case the deafness was diagnosed during the course of the illness, at approximately the end of the first week, and steroids were given deliberately. No conclusions are being drawn, but the facts are mentioned for the reader's interest.

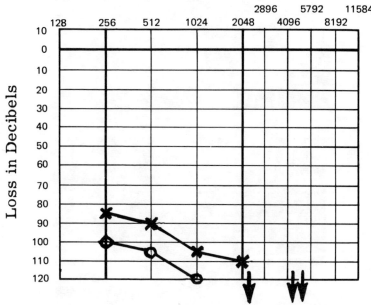

Figure 32   Typical post-meningitic hearing loss: air conduction; ○ right ear, × left ear; no bone conduction recorded

One other point should be made about the treatment of meningitis. Some years ago the usual triad treatment of chloramphenicol, penicillin and sulphonamide was altered to treatment with ampicillin alone. It was then found necessary to use very large doses, 300–400 mg/kg per day, divided into four to six intravenous doses[2] to avoid failures in some cases due to *Haemophilus influenzae*. Following this change a report followed from Sweden[3] that from 1971 to 1972 at least fourteen out of around 400 children treated in this way had developed bilateral severe sensorineural hearing loss. This caused paediatricians to consider whether ampicillin alone was either ineffective as treatment for

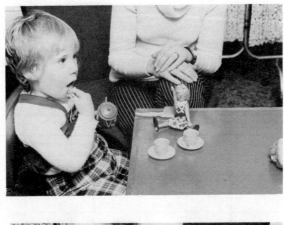

(a)

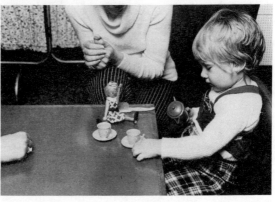

(b)

Figures 33 (a) and (b)   Child of 18 months, profoundly deaf
following meningitis, but showing normal 'inner language'
or symbolic play

meningitis, or whether it was indeed another ototoxic drug.
However subsequent work done by Jones and Hanson[4]
seemed to prove reasonably conclusively that it was only
when ampicillin was given in doses *exceeding* 250 mg/kg per
day that there was a true correlation between its administration and subsequent sensorineural hearing loss. It does,
therefore, seem very probable that ampicillin in very large

doses is ototoxic, and the treatment of choice in most cases of meningitis remains chloramphenicol, penicillin and sulphonamide.

Measles and mumps

Measles and mumps, as mentioned above, occasionally cause sensorineural deafness as a complication. Although this is usually a unilateral hearing loss it is not to be taken lightly, as it can prove a problem in the classroom and later on at work or at social gatherings. The unilateral deafness is usually very severe, and often referred to as 'a dead ear' because of the very small amount of hearing remaining.

Minor conductive hearing losses

Lastly we must again mention the minor conductive hearing losses of childhood. In testing very young babies it is not at all unusual to find them responding at 50 dB rather than the acceptable screening level of 40 dB. Also it is often quite noticeable that their response to the Manchester or Nuffield rattle is much brisker than that to the cup and spoon, which contains low frequency elements. Their tympanic membranes already appear dull and, in fact, they are giving the typical signs of secretory otitis media. Parents often report that they have been 'snuffly since birth'. It is our practice to keep such babies under observation, so that suitable help can be offered at the right time (see Chapter 15). Of course these findings become even more common as the child gets older, with a longer history of upper respiratory tract infections and, possibly, but not always, frank ear infections. It is very important to remember how commonly conductive hearing loss occurs in early childhood, up to around the age of 6–7 years, when the incidence lessens markedly. Remember, again, that the small, recurrent, conductive hearing loss is very important indeed, and can severely affect the normal development of language or acquisition of reading skills. This subject is dealt with fully in Chapter 15.

References

1. Keleman (1963). Quoted by Fraser, Chap 12, p. 248

2. Fenwick, J.D. (1975). Neonatal jaundice as a cause of deafness. *Laryngol. Otol.*, **89**, 925

3. Gamstorp, I. and Hanson, D.R. (1974). Hearing loss after *H. influenzae* meningitis. *Devel. Med. Child Neurol.*, **16**, 678–679

4. Jones, F. E. and Hanson, D. R. (1977). *Devel. Med. Child Neurol.*, **19**, 593–597

Chapter 13

THE TREATMENT OF SENSORINEURAL HEARING LOSS
(a) AMPLIFICATION

The first step in the treatment of sensorineural hearing loss is, of course, its diagnosis. This is why we lay such stress on the regular examination of infants and children, on the accuracy of the tests used, and on the ability of the examiner to interpret his test results correctly. Congenital hearing loss should be diagnosed within the first year of life and a baby should be using amplification comfortably by its first birthday, or by the time it learns to walk.

The treatment of sensorineural hearing loss can be divided into three sections dealt with in this Chapter and Chapter 14:

(1) The prescription of amplification suitable for the child's hearing loss.

(2) Good auditory training, commencing at the moment of diagnosis.

(3) At a later stage, the choice of correct educational placement for the child.

USE OF AMPLIFICATION

This subject could, in itself, take a whole volume, but here only the basic essentials of a hearing aid are described.

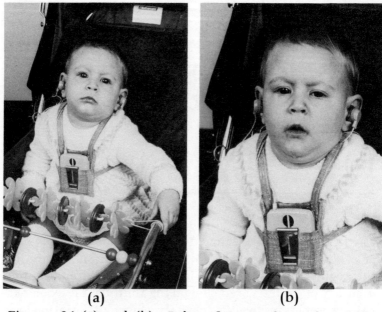

(a)   (b)

Figures 34 (a) and (b) Baby of 9 months with rubella hearing loss, using hearing aid. Note that he is already learning to use the aid consistently; (a) shows him in his pram 'going shopping' with his mother

An enormous range of hearing aids are manufactured. The manufacturer supplies, with his aid, graphs to show both how much amplification is given at each frequency, and also the total sound output of the aid. It is therefore the task of the audiologist or otologist to 'match up' the hearing loss of the patient against the amplification produced by the aid and choose the most appropriate one.

Hearing aids are basically of two types – the body-worn aid and the postaural aid. Until recently only body-worn aids were really adequate for the child with a severe hearing loss; now, however, with the rapid advances in electronics, very high-powered postaural aids are available.

What are the 'pros and cons' of the two types? Firstly in a very young baby postaural aids are not suitable, as they are easily pulled out by a determined baby and thrown into quite irretrievable positions – for example, a baby in his pram may have his postaural aid under a passing bus before his mother can take preventive action. The age at which postaural aids become practicable depends very much upon the child. I have had a little girl aged 16 months using postaural aids with complete success, but I would say that this is, in general, too young to try them. There are also some 2-year-olds who can manage them very competently, but on the whole 3 years is probably the minimum age they should be considered for the child with a moderate hearing loss. There are several advantages of the postaural aid. First of all sound reaches the child from *all* directions, instead of only entering the microphone from the front, a much more 'natural' way of receiving sound input. Those lucky enough to have two normally hearing ears receive sound from all around and this is more nearly imitated, although not exactly, by the postaural aid. It is important to note the position of the microphone on any postaural aid. Most now are on the front of the aid, which seems to give best results.

In addition the young child wearing two postaural aids gains a good deal more freedom than a child using two body-worn aids. It is easier for the child to run, jump, climb, roll on the grass, etc. than its peer encumbered with two biggish 'boxes' secured in a harness on its chest. This was pointed out to me very firmly by the eminently sensible mother of a 3-year-old. She said that the difference in her daughter's possible activities, and therefore in her life, was remarkable. Critics will probably remark that body-worn aids can be removed during very vigorous active play, and this of course is quite true, so parents of children using body-worn aids are always advised about this fact. There are, of course, some activities where removal of any aid is necessary for both safety and comfort. However, in those cases, for instance, where the normal 3-year-old is engaging in normal play in the garden, it is much more satisfactory if he can retain his aids in position, so that as he plays he can also communicate with his companions. In addition, in active play he is not disturbed by the rub of his clothes against the microphone of the aids.

Lastly, and this *is* a very important point, there is the question of 'cosmetics'. Most parents, already heartbroken by the discovery that their beautiful baby has a severe hearing loss, may even become near-hysterical when they realize that he is to be encumbered with two body-worn hearing aids on his chest. Of course it is explained to them, with the greatest care and sympathy, that the aids are to help him hear, so that he may develop as much speech as possible. However, for the parents of a 9-month-old baby in the middle of the emotional turmoil caused by the diagnosis, these logical arguments may carry little weight at that stage. Their feelings are, quite understandably, that a tragedy has happened, their child is 'different' and they wish to conceal and hide the evidence of this 'differentness' as far as they possibly can. It is almost as if they feel that by hiding the evidence they can make it all go away. At this point very careful parent counselling is necessary, for no parents can really begin to help their child until they have accepted, and come to terms with, his handicap. Accepting the necessity of the hearing aids, particularly body-worn aids, is part of the much larger problem of accepting the child's hearing loss as a whole, with all its implications.

In many cases the parents have the consolation of knowing that as the child becomes older body-worn aids can be exchanged for postaural aids, and with recent technological advances, this is becoming true for more and more children.

So far we have talked about the feelings of the parents towards the aids. But now we must mention the young patients themselves, with their feelings and problems of

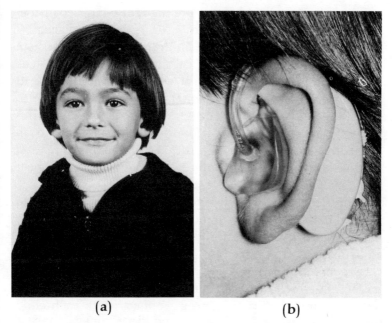

(a)   (b)

Figures 35 (a) and (b)   A very handsome 6-year-old, using postaural aids which are completely hidden; (b) shows the aid, with its mould, in close-up view

'differentness'. There comes a stage in the life of every severely deaf boy or girl when, having happily used body-worn aids for many years, he or she suddenly 'demands' postaural aids. In some cases, unfortunately all too frequently, children wear their aids *only* in school and when under direct supervision. Immediately they are out of the classroom their body-worn aids are discarded, and few parents insist that they should be replaced. Thus many older children spend every evening, weekend, and twelve weeks of school holiday without amplification. No wonder their speech is minimal! They communicate, albeit often very adequately, by a mixture of single words, very poorly enunciated, plus their own complicated gestural system. But such a method, adequate for the moment, is totally inadequate for anything much more than the simple cognitive processes. However, if the body-worn aids are replaced by suitable postaural aids such children normally use them consistently, for when postaural aids are hidden by hair their 'differentness' is reduced at a stroke. In an ideal world all children above a certain mental age would have access to postaural aids carefully selected for their particular requirements, to radio-linked aids for the classroom, and to an alternative system of communication to aid their acquisition of spoken language. More will be said about the latter aspect in Chapter 14.

Many teachers, however, still prefer body-worn aids to be used in the classroom. Whichever type is used, however, it is essential that they be fitted with the necessary adjustment for connection to the loop system in the classroom or to the television at home. This loop system is a method in which the classroom is wired so that the teacher speaking into a microphone can 'connect' with each child directly, via his or her aid. The child can answer into a microphone which again connects back to his aid, so that he can hear the sound of his own voice. Obviously this is very important when the teacher is working on such matters as intonation and articulation. So it is immediately apparent that a postaural aid *without* a loop setting is useless for a child attending a school or unit with looped classrooms and it also deprives him of the value of a loop fitted into the television set. There are also some churches, theatres and cinemas fitted with a loop system for the convenience of deaf people in the audience.

In addition to this some teachers prefer the sound to go into the microphone on the front of the child because of the way in which the classroom is arranged. If the children are sitting in a crescent around the teacher then obviously more sound will go from the teacher into microphones worn on the front of the child. This, of course, applies particularly to formal academic classroom situations and not to the sort of lesson in which the child is actively moving while he works, such as projects, craft, art, etc. As more and more work is done via project systems tailored to individual needs, the need for body-worn aids diminishes. In some schools and units children are able to wear body-worn aids for very formal work and postaural aids for all other situations.

I think it must be stressed, however, that postaural aids have improved so vastly that shortly very few children will need to use body-worn aids. Preliminary experiments with selected very young children have been highly successful.

The body-worn aid consists of the main 'box' containing the amplifier and the microphone, the receiver head (or earpiece) containing, as its name implies, the receiver and the lead connecting the two (Figure 36). The receiver head clips into the 'mould' which fits snugly into the patient's ear. If the mould does not fit well (perhaps because of wax in the ear which should be removed before making a new mould) then a distressing whistle is produced when the aid is switched on or the volume switched up. In children the size of the ear alters so rapidly in growth, that moulds may need to be remade at very frequent intervals. *It must be stressed that if the mould is not made well and does not fit really well then the expensive aid is totally wasted.* This puts a heavy responsibility on technicians who make the moulds, particularly in the case of young children who are often not the easiest of patients to handle over this matter.

The technician must take an impression of the child's ear by gently pushing plastic silicone material into the child's ear. A hardening agent is added to get an impression which maintains its shape. (The child often enjoys playing with a piece of the material while this is being done, as it bears some resemblance to plasticine.) He waits a few minutes for the impression to 'set' and the material is then removed from the child's ear. The technician is now left with a 'model' of the shape of the interior of the pinna and the first part of the external auditory canal. This is trimmed to make a neat exact

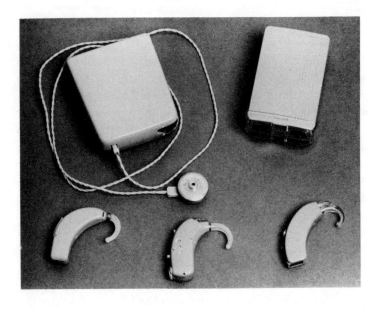

Figure 36   The body-worn aid on the left is the OL56, specially manufactured for use in the National Health Service. The microphone is on the reverse side, but can be clearly seen on the baby in Figures 34(a) and (b). The body-worn aid on the right is a commercial aid which is extremely powerful, and used only for children with profound hearing loss. The single aid is unusual in being manufactured specially to give amplification to *both* ears, that is the child only needs to use one instead of two aids (note the microphone at the top of the aid). The postaural aid on the left is the BE11, again specially manufactured for use in the National Health Service. Both the OL56 and the BE11 are suitable for patients with only a moderate hearing loss. The postaural aid on the right is bought under government contract and is more powerful than the BE11. The middle postaural aid is specific for high-frequency loss and can be set, via four controls, to suit an individual's loss in the higher frequencies, *without* amplifying the low frequencies

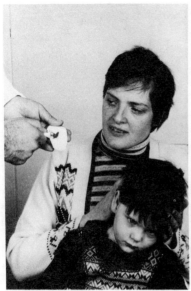

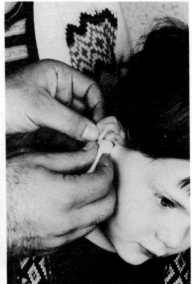

Fig 37a

Fig 37b

Fig 37c

Fig 37d

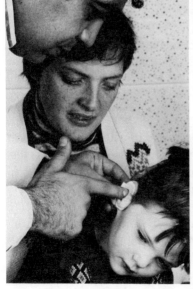

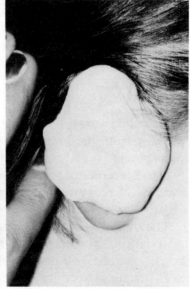

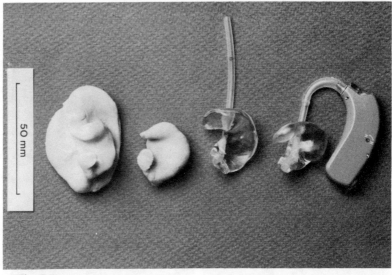

Fig 37e

Figure 37   Making a mould. (a) Adding hardener to the silicone material; they are thoroughly mixed by rolling in the fingers. (b) Putting the prepared material into the ear. (c) Pressing the material gently into the ear. (d) Allowing the mould to 'set' in the ear for 2 to 3 minutes. (e) From the left: the mould removed from the ear; the mould after trimming, ready to be sent to the factory; the mould returned from the factory, ready for use; the mould attached to the postaural aid

model, and then sent off to the factory where the final mould is made from the impression using a plaster of paris cast. Incorporated in the mould is one half of the stud which fixes it to the receiver head (see Figure 36). A stud is not used in the case of postaural aids, where tubing is substituted (see Figure 37(e)).

The final mould may be made of different types of plastic material. It may be a so-called 'hard' mould, made of hard acrylic material which is tough and difficult to break, or 'soft', made of soft acrylic material which gives a greater degree of comfort but may more easily lose shape and fitting. The best type is probably the harder mould with a soft tip, which hopefully combines the advantages of both. There are, however, many different materials that can be used, and very often a material that suits one person is totally unsuitable for another; for instance, some people are allergic to almost all the commonly used materials and require a very special non-allergic material such as vulcanite. If this is not used they develop an otitis externa which can be difficult to treat.

In the body-worn aid used with a receiver head, not only must the aid be chosen to suit the patient's loss but it must also be remembered that the receiver head can alter the final amplification received by the patient. Thus when a hearing aid is prescribed for any patient, the receiver head required to go with the aid must also be clearly stated.

In the postaural aid the amplifier, receiver and micro-phone are all incorporated into the same small body. A fine piece of tubing leads from the aid into the specially made mould, which again must fit snugly into the ear (see Figure 37(e)). It cannot be stressed too much that many children are unable to use expensive, powerful aids to their full advantage because moulds have not been made carefully. I have met many parents who have told me that they could not turn the aid past volume 1 or 2, because of the whistling, when the required amplification was probably at least at volume 6. Whenever possible, it is worth removing wax before moulds are made, thus cutting out at least one troublesome factor.

Many people, unfamiliar with the use of hearing aids, think that the whistling sound means that the aid itself is faulty, but this is rarely the case. It is advisable to check first the fit of the moulds and then the auditory canals for wax.

The Department of Health has laid down the principle that every *child* with a hearing loss shall have prescribed for its use that aid which is most suitable for its needs.

Otologists and audiologists are asked to prescribe those aids, which are manufactured specifically for use in National Health Service hospitals and clinics, whenever *these are suitable* for the patient. They are also asked to prescribe those commercial aids, bought under government contract, in a similar way, that is whenever they are suitable for the individual patient under consideration. If the patient's needs are *not* covered by these aids, and the patient is under 18 years of age, or in full-time education up to the age of 21 years, then the specialist may prescribe *any aid which he considers will give maximum benefit to the patient*. This, unfortunately, does not apply to the third type of aid, which we have only briefly mentioned so far.

The radio-linked aid

In the radio-linked aid, as the name implies, there is a direct radio link between the child and either the parent or teacher or other partner in the conversation. The parent or teacher wears the microphone, while the child wears the receiver, and there is a direct link whether the child is close at hand, in another room or even outside in the garden. The instrument also incorporates 'compression' which means that the aid automatically fails to amplify very loud sounds, thus cutting out the distress which this can sometimes cause to many deaf patients. (In fact 'compression' is steadily being introduced into more and more aids of all types.)

The radio-linked aid produces direct connection between speaker and listener, cutting out extraneous noise that would normally also be amplified and interfere badly with the amplification of speech and its reception by the listener. This, of course, is the primary fault of all other hearing aids. They not only amplify the speech which is so vital to the deaf child, but also all the other sounds which, so to speak, 'surround' the speech. Normally hearing people can easily pick out speech from among the welter of domestic or classroom sounds that may be going on simultaneously. But if *all* are amplified for the deaf child his task at separating out the essential speech sounds from the non-essential background noise is made very difficult. This is done for him by a direct radio link.

As mentioned above, in an ideal world the deaf child would have access to this type of amplification. The problem is, of course, the cost of the apparatus, which is between £700 and £800, at the time of writing.* Many parents make very brave attempts to save up the amount of money required, some of them even saving their attendance allowance for this purpose. In many parts of the United Kingdom, education departments are realizing the enormous value of radio-link apparatus, and are providing this as part of their educational service for the deaf.

The only other type of aid which cannot be prescribed for children under the National Health Service, is the spectacle frame which also incorporates the aid in its arm. Many adults, however, find this type of aid convenient and worth the considerable financial outlay.

---

* Aids of this type include the Jessop Aid, the Radio Link Aid (Shulberg) and the Phonic Ear (P.C. Werth).

Chapter 14

THE TREATMENT OF SENSORINEURAL HEARING LOSS
(b) AUDITORY TRAINING AND SPECIAL EDUCATION

In Chapter 13 it was stated that the treatment of the deaf child consists of three main parts:

(1) Good, suitable amplification.
(2) Auditory training, from the moment of diagnosis.
(3) Suitable educational placement at the right age.

This chapter deals with parts (2) and (3), auditory training, and special education.

AUDITORY TRAINING

The normal hearing baby vocalizes from birth. By the age of 4 weeks or so a happy, contented infant is producing cooing and gurgling sounds. It is a great pity that more parents do not listen actively to their newly born infants to hear these sounds – vowel or low-frequency sounds – which are really quite delightful in nature.

At the age of 3–4 months the infant's vocalizations change to produce babbling sounds, which contain high-frequency notes. At 6 months the normal baby produces a lovely babbled conversation either in response to an adult's overtures or when he is happily settled in his cot. The deaf baby, however, although he often produces the low-frequency cooing and gurgling sounds, fails at 3–4 months to change the nature of his vocalization. In other words, as he is often unable to hear the high-frequency sounds, he cannot reproduce them. Mothers very often notice that their deaf baby's vocalizations are unlike those of older, normal siblings at the same age. Sometimes deaf babies are said to be 'very quiet' producing very few vocalizations other than crying. On the other hand they may be quite noisy, but the 'noise' they produce is quite unlike the tuneful vocalizations of the baby with normal hearing. Of course if the deaf baby is also a first baby then the mother has not the advantage of comparison (which, on the whole, is usually to be deplored, but this is one instance when it can be useful).

With the normal hearing baby, at around the age of 1 year, the babbled Dad-dad-dad becomes meaningful for 'Daddy' and gradually other babble sounds are replaced by consistent sounds which have meaning for the child, even if the sound is not entirely the same as the word used by an adult to describe the object. This stage coincides with another very important developmental landmark. At the age of 9 months, if a small baby's hairbrush is given to him he explores it in quite a thorough manner, with hands, eyes and mouth, before he drops it. However, by the age of 12–14 months the hairbrush has acquired further significance for the child, and when it is handed to him he usually puts it up to his hair, in brief imitation of how he has seen it used. In other words he is 'defining by use' (see Chapter 7). He shows the same change when given a cup; instead of investigating it as he did at 9 months, when probably his chief pleasure was to bang it on any hard surface available, thus producing a loud, satisfactory noise, he now puts it up to his mouth in a very purposeful way. Again he is 'defining by use'. Thus the two parameters of development proceed, so to speak, hand in hand. Babble sounds, previously used for vocal play, begin to achieve a meaning. Objects, previously used for exploratory play, begin to achieve a meaningful use. The hearing child goes on to acquire a small vocabulary of nouns by the age of 18 months. These are followed by adjectives and verbs, so that at the age of 2–2$\frac{1}{4}$ years he can join words, first subject–verb or verb–object constructions, and then at around 2$\frac{1}{2}$ subject–verb–object constructions.

The child with a hearing loss, however, can only proceed along *one* of these parameters, that is he shows 'definition by use' at the same stage as his hearing peer. But, as we have already said, he probably cannot produce any babble and his first words do not appear at the expected time. If the loss is only very moderate he may produce a few words at a much later stage, with poor intelligibility. If he has a high frequency loss he may produce a normal quantity of vocalization but this is intelligible to no-one except himself.

As well as producing expressive language the normal baby, from around the age of 1 year, also begins to acquire more and more verbal comprehension. Thus, by 18 months, as we have seen in Chapter 9, the child is able to hand a few simple objects on request, selecting the correct one from a line of around five toys and common objects placed in front of him, such as a brush, a cup, a spoon, a toy car, and a doll.

The child with a hearing loss, although he understands the function of the objects in front of him, and can demonstrate their use quite correctly, is totally unable to pick them out by name. He differs from a mentally retarded child who can neither hand the objects by name *nor* demonstrate their use. At this stage the latter is probably still mouthing and casting the objects, thus showing quite different behaviour from that of the normally intelligent deaf child.

If then, we diagnose a hearing loss in a baby by the age of 9 months (which should always be the aim), provide suitable amplification for that baby, we then have to consider the enormous task of *teaching* it all the stages of speech which the normal baby acquires so easily and effortlessly, provided that he is receiving normal stimulation in a caring home.

One of the first stages is to show the baby that there is an interesting and fascinating world of sound going on around him. His interest must be aroused by presenting him with varieties of auditory stimuli, which he can hear with his aids *in situ*. These stimuli may be many and varied, ranging from patterns of sound made on a drum or xylophone, through all sorts of musical sounds, going on to the interesting domestic sounds, such as water running into his bath, the sound of the vacuum cleaner, washing machine, food mixer, etc., or the sounds of his siblings or other children shouting as they play, and the outdoor sounds of traffic, trains, etc. Combined with all these must be the sounds of his parents' voices, talking to him in a simple meaningful way.

Obviously there is a great deal of information to be given to the parents about how they must tackle the enormous task that lies ahead. This is the responsibility of the *peripatetic* or *visiting teacher of the deaf*, who is alerted, via the local Education Department, directly the diagnosis of hearing loss is made. She visits as soon as possible, and this first visit to the parents is of crucial importance. She may often find the parents in a state of extreme shock and distress, often amounting to despair. They may query the diagnosis, they may want to have a second opinion, and they will have many, many questions to be answered. Will he talk? Will he get worse? Is there a cure? Must he wear hearing aids? What sort of hearing aids can he have? Can we buy him 'better' hearing aids? What school will he be able to attend? It needs all the skill, tact, patience and expertise of the teacher to guide the parents through this extremely difficult period and bring them slowly but surely to the acceptance of the child's handicap. It is often easier for parents to accept the situation if they realize how much they have to do and how much the future of their child depends largely on their efforts, which must commence immediately.

As already mentioned above the child must be introduced to the fascinating world of sound, and if the sounds are interesting then the baby begins to *listen*. This eventually leads him to listen to his mother's and his father's voices, and then try to reproduce some of what he is hearing for the first time. So at this stage we hope he will begin to babble, or produce sounds which are not merely noises but contain speech sounds including consonants.

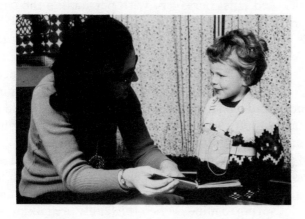

Figure 38 The peripatetic teacher of the deaf at work

It is really the job of the teacher of the deaf to instruct and guide parents so that *they* become the teachers of their child, with advice and help geared to the individual needs of their child's particular problems.

The teacher helps the parents to realize that each new step must be encouraged, praised and rewarded, so that the young child is encouraged to repeat it. 'Rewards' in this context does not mean that every new piece of babble should be greeted with a sweet or piece of chocolate, but rather that the parents should smile, hug, and show obvious pleasure to the child. All human beings thrive on appropriate praise, even the very young child. The teacher also explains to the parents the importance of the child not only hearing sounds but also seeing them on the lips of the parents. Many children, who have an undiagnosed hearing loss, learn to lip-read spontaneously, at a very early age. Children, in fact, seem to vary quite widely in their ability to learn to lip-read. But in the same way that they have to be taught to 'listen' they also have to be taught to 'look'. The child who has, in addition, any sort of attention problem, also finds 'looking', in a sustained way, very difficult. But all concerned must persevere with persuading the child to look while he listens.

It is obviously very important for parents to talk to the child a very great deal. But it is of little value to talk to the child as if holding a conversation with another hearing adult. The parents must use rather short, meaningful sentences, and *not* shout. Whenever possible the child must be in a position to see the words being used. (Obviously there are exceptions to this on many occasions, such as when driving a car, but it is a rule that should be used at *all* appropriate times.) The parents must also show the child the meaning of the words being used, as far as possible. Many examples spring to mind. When the family are talking about driving the car, then the child must be shown the car, and also his toy car, while he hears the word *car* and sees the shape of the word *car* on his parents' lips. Thus, as the child slowly progresses, with the parents using the same common and important words time and time again, he can slowly begin to build a vocabulary of nouns. These are usually words to do with everyday routines, which his parents have said to him, have shown to him on their lips and have associated with the real object.

Obviously it is quite useless for a child to build up a vocabulary of words which he does not comprehend; but this can happen when parents merely insist that a child repeats a word after them, without any reference to the meaning of the word. Thus, it is quite useless for a parent to sit down with a child and then ask him to say *car, cup, spoon,* etc. The child may well learn to echo *car, cup* and *spoon,* but unless these exercises are combined with reference to a real car, a real cup and a real spoon, then the parents are merely producing 'a parrot'. The same thing may happen at a much later stage when the child learns to read, which he may do quite fluently, in a mechanical fashion, but with very little comprehension of what he is saying. Thus teachers are always extremely careful to ensure that each passage read has also been fully comprehended. The rule with any child, hearing or deaf, must be that *comprehension precedes expression.*

When the child has built up a useful vocabulary of nouns he can probably begin to learn some adjectives. It is quite easy to illustrate opposite adjectives, such as big and little, hot and cold, etc., and at the same time the names of colours. All the time each word is patiently learned by sound, by the appearance on the lips of the speaker, and by reference to the object, to illustrations, models, etc.

Probably at around this time the child is also learning the meaning of simple prepositions, such as *in, on* and *under.* Again all of these are easily illustrated to the child and are usually learnt quite readily when the teacher is competent. The work becomes harder as the prepositions become more complicated. A simple example illustrates the type of difficulty encountered at an early stage: the difference between *behind* and *beside.* To the reader this may seem an easily illustrated difference, but for the young deaf child the teacher and parents must patiently persist in demonstrating the difference at all possible times until the concept has become firmly established and connected with both the sounds and shapes of the words.

At this stage, then, the child may have a reasonably good naming vocabulary, know a few adjectives and also the commonest prepositions, usually *in* and *on* because these are used so frequently by all the family. But now the child reaches the most difficult step, the use of verbs. In normal conversation how often does one consider whether to use the present tense, the present continuous, the past perfect, the past imperfect or even the future? When this is carefully considered it is apparent how enormous is the problem confronting the severely deaf child. It is little wonder that many of these children, even at the age of 14 years or so, have to be coaxed into using verbs when communicating. But if the child is to develop its cognitive abilities it is essential that it learns how to use verbs at the earliest possible time. The use of the verb is a big landmark in the 'learning life' of the deaf child, and at the same time it probably presents the biggest stumbling block. It is because of this, that when I hear the child using its first subject–verb or verb–object constructions I feel the parent–teacher–child team has fulfilled a major task and I share their delight and pleasure in the achievement.

The next logical step is for the child to put together the subject–verb and verb–object constructions to produce a subject–verb–object utterance. By this stage teacher and parents have laid the enormously important foundation and it is upon this foundation that they can continue to build, patiently and slowly.

We must never underestimate the problems. How, for instance, do you explain to your severely deaf child that he has to go to the dentist, to go into hospital, to stay with a friend while *you* keep a hospital appointment? How do you explain 'tomorrow', or that his grandmother, perhaps dearly loved, has died? The reader can probably think immediately of dozens of similar examples.

However, as the complexity of the child's language increases the same rules must be observed. The parent and teacher much continually ensure that his verbal comprehension is as good as his verbal expression. Our aim must be to produce a child who is both able to use and understand complex sentences, with clauses, a child who has a sound understanding of our highly complicated English syntax, and above all a child who is able to express his thoughts, in spoken language, intelligible to those around him. This *must* be our aim, although to many of us dealing with hundreds of deaf children it tends to sound a wildly improbable dream.

We have not, so far, spoken of articulatory problems, which are obviously worse in those children with a severe high-frequency loss. Unfortunately even our very best hearing aids perform worst in the high frequencies. So there must be many deaf children who never hear the high-frequency consonants and who have to rely upon lip-reading alone in attempting to reproduce such consonants as *s* and *s* blends, *th*, *f*, etc. (see Figure 2 in Chapter 3).

With very young deaf children the initial aim must be to produce vocalizations, then babble, and then word approximations. While the child is learning this and also the next steps of noun vocabulary and the early word-joining constructions, it is much more important to encourage his flow of speech rather than to correct his articulation. A young child, constantly corrected for articulatory errors, stands a very real chance of ceasing his efforts. He may, very easily 'dry up' and be pushed back into being both non-communicative and probably very frustrated again. Therefore, the initial aim must be to produce the language, while the articulation work can be done when the teacher judges it to be appropriate.

The peripatetic teacher has another piece of equipment which will be a great help to both parents and child through the long struggle to acquire language. This is known as a *speech trainer* and is an instrument where the teacher speaks into a microphone and the child hears the amplified sound directly through earphones (Figure 39). The child also has a microphone into which he can speak and thus hear his own voice. This ability to hear his *own* vocalizations is very important for the deaf child, and the earlier he can hear them, the better are his chances of acquiring some reasonable speech. It is very important always to remember that the deaf child may hear very little of his own voice, hence the value of the speech trainer and, later in school, the group aid with individual microphones.

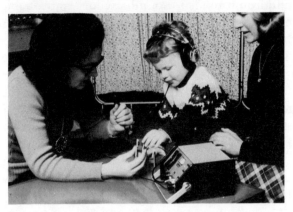

Figure 39   The use of the speech trainer

The age at which the speech trainer is tolerated varies widely and the teacher must usually judge the right moment from her own experience. Some children of 18 months use it for repeated, *very short*, periods, while others do not tolerate it until nearer 3 years. Obviously a very active child does not want to sit for long periods with the head-phones *in situ*. So the ingenuity of parents and teacher must produce situations of great interest connected with speech trainer sessions. At a very much later stage the speech trainer can be used to improve articulation.

We have shown that the postdiagnostic, preschool period is of crucial importance. There is no doubt that early diagnosis, with adequate amplification immediately, and with skilled peripatetic teaching help coupled with parental enthusiasm and determination, influences the final outcome enormously.

However, it would be very wrong to leave the reader with the impression that if one fulfils all these criteria the prognosis for speech is good. Unhappily, this is not the complete picture. Obviously when the loss is profound then the prognosis is worse. If the loss is subsequent to meningitis then other areas may also have been damaged. If the loss seems to have been associated with problems in pregnancy or perinatal problems again other areas may have been damaged. (I am not referring here to children so grossly damaged that they show the picture of mental subnormality with deafness and possibly also with cerebral palsy.) But there are many children with normal performance IQs who appear to have all the advantages, and yet do not develop language at the expected rate. Conversely we see, from time to time, children who show the opposite picture. These, perhaps, have not been diagnosed until the age of 3 years and have received very little preschool help and yet, once the help is provided, they progress at a most surprising rate. Such contrasting children have caused considerable discussion in our clinics, and posed many questions.

I think the answer possibly lies in concurrent damage that some children may suffer, quite specifically, in the language areas of the brain, in addition to the damage that has been done, and can be demonstrated to occur, in the localized region of the cochlea. While this sort of answer is very feasible when deafness occurs as a result of a potentially generalized damaging factor it does not logically explain the differences that seem to occur in the progress of children with genetically determined deafness. There is, as mentioned above, scope for much more research in this area, and these points only reinforce this necessity.

There is still no doubt that to give any deaf child the best chance of producing the results that are optimal for him we must have early diagnosis, early and adequate amplification, with immediate effective preschool help in auditory training. The latter must be produced by a strong cooperative partnership of advisory, peripatetic teacher of the deaf and the whole family of the hearing-handicapped child.

THE TIME FOR SCHOOL

Every education authority has a duty to provide special education for a handicapped child from the age of $2\frac{1}{2}$ years. It seems that, in the case of deaf children, this duty is interpreted by different authorities in many different ways. Some continue to provide a visiting teacher until the child is almost 5 years of age, before transferring his care to a formal school. In the meantime the child is usually placed in a normal-hearing playgroup on an increasing number of days. While this can be taken as fulfilling 'the letter of the law' it is certainly insufficient for most deaf children to make optimal progress, especially when it is remembered that a deaf child is very lucky if it has two 1 hour sessions weekly with its teacher (one such weekly session is much more likely). Exposure to a group of normally hearing children, on a frequent regular basis, when the deaf child can understand very little language and can certainly not use expressive language in any way approaching that of the group, can be very harmful to many deaf children. They become more and more frustrated, excluded and 'different', and this is quickly shown in their behaviour. They cannot understand instructions, but have to search for situational clues to follow the group. They find it very hard to learn 'socialization' when the basis of this is learning to communicate, and this they cannot do. Such pleasures as singing games can only be copied, without being understood; the end-of-session story isolates them to the maximum degree. No wonder they come home and indulge in a major temper tantrum.

This type of provision is only suitable for the child with a mild-to-moderate loss, who is making very good progress, whose teacher visits him in the playgroup as well as at home, whose parents provide a good back-up to the playgroup activities which may not have been understood by the child, who is being prepared for entry to a normal school with continuing peripatetic help.

This is, in fact, the first type of special educational help that may be offered to a child with a hearing loss, in other words he may be able to attend a normal school with regular visits from his peripatetic teacher of the deaf, who ensures that the amplification is used and understood by his class teacher. The hearing aid itself must be checked regularly, to ensure that it is working adequately, moulds checked and the provision of new ones arranged whenever necessary. Apart from these technical points the child's progress is discussed with the staff who teach him, and who find it hard to understand the difficulties faced by the deaf child in a hearing world. It is the job of the teacher of the deaf to 'educate' her colleagues, acquainting them with the common problems of deafness, and to alert them to situations where difficulties commonly arise.

There is the question of the deaf child who reads fluently but understands only a small part of what he reads. There is the question of the child with a high-frequency hearing loss, where even experienced teachers may deny his deafness until his audiogram is seen and understood. Only then do some teachers change a label from 'dreamy', 'inattentive', 'lacking in concentration', 'naughty', or even 'disturbed', to that of 'deaf'. This of course can change the whole nature of the child's subsequent educational career, progress and even life, as he may no longer be viewed as a troublemaker but rather as a child with a handicap to treat. The ensuing difference in the teacher's attitude can, finally, be met by a corresponding improvement in the child's behaviour pattern. Nobody pretends that it happens overnight, but given a teacher who now understands the handicap and the symptoms, and is well motivated to help, then quite surely there are bound to be gradual improvements in terms of both behaviour and educational achievement.

Sometimes the deaf child in an ordinary class meets a 'sticking point' where even special help from his class teacher is insufficient. Some classes are still so large that the teacher is unable to give all the extra time that he or she would like to spend with the deaf child. Here, then, is another area where the visiting teacher may well be able to help, perhaps with a certain stage of arithmetic, where the child's language has failed him and he has missed an important basic concept. The teacher herself may well provide some extra help and time to put this right or may discuss methods with his class teacher to help him grasp a particular idea which is holding up progress. The progress of a deaf child in a hearing class may well be radically improved by the use of any of the radio-link apparatuses, where they are particularly suitable (see Chapter 13).

If the child's hearing loss is such that he requires many hours of special help, or special apparatus such as the auditory trainer or the group aid, but is nevertheless making a lot of progress with speech, then the ideal school placement is a partially hearing unit contained within a normal school (Figure 40). The child can then have a programme geared to his particular needs. He can spend as much time in the unit as the teacher deems appropriate because the unit is staffed by specially trained and experienced teachers. His own apparatus can be checked daily, and he can use it in the unit to whatever extent is necessary. On the other hand he can spend increasing amounts of time in an ordinary class. At first this may only be for lessons such as PE, dancing, games or art, but this can then be extended as the child's progress allows until, ideally, he spends almost all his school life in the ordinary class, returning to the unit only to have his apparatus checked or when he needs special help over a difficult concept. The unit, however, is always there as a safeguard and back-up system which gives confidence to staff and child alike. Perhaps even more importantly, the child with a

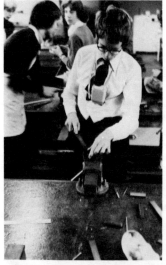

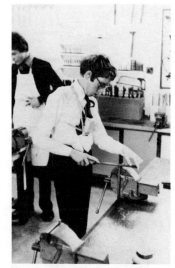

Fig 40a

Fig 40b

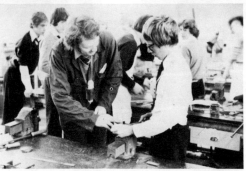

Fig 40c

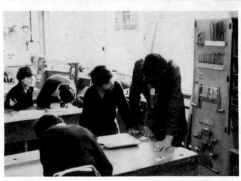

Fig 40d

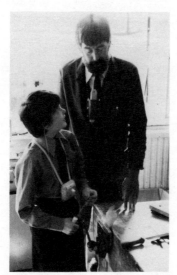

Fig 40e

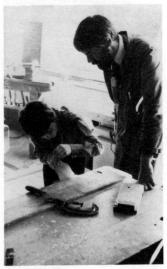

Fig 40f

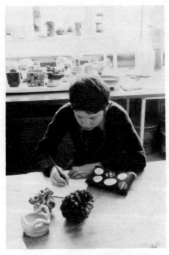

Fig 40g

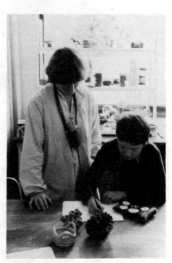

Fig 40h

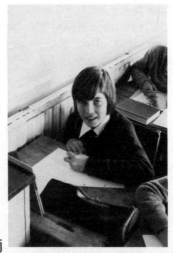

Fig 40j

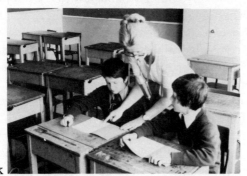

Fig 40k

Figure 40   Boys in a partially hearing unit, illustrating the use of radio-linked apparatus. (a) and (b) Partially hearing twins, in the metalwork department. (c) Note the teacher's use of the microphone. (d), (e) and (f) Using the equipment in the woodwork department. (g) and (h) Use of radio-link equipment in the pottery department. (j) Partially hearing pupil can join a normal 'academic' group with this apparatus. (k) Extra help is at hand if necessary, in a big school, with a small unit involved as part of that school

hearing loss eats and plays with his hearing peers, which is of tremendous benefit to both sides. The hearing child who has grown up alongside deaf colleagues is far less likely to turn into the objectionable adult for whom 'deafness' is equated with 'dimness'.

If the child, however, has such a serious loss or is making extremely slow progress with speech, then his educational treatment needs to be even more specialized and he is usually admitted to a school for the deaf. At the moment such schools tend to fall into two groups. First, those who persist with oral methods of communication at all costs, regardless of the slowness of the process, maintaining that 'signing' is the easy way out and that children who sign will never speak. They back up their attitudes by pointing out that the 'deaf' child has got to live in a 'hearing' world, and that signing may only push him back into the enclosed little world of other deaf people, their families, teachers and friends, who can also 'sign'. Second, the other group of schools which teach oral methods *combined* with a signing or manual system. There are now no schools at all where emphasis is laid *only* on signing.

It is my own very strongly held belief that the optimal treatment for this group of children is a basically oral approach, plus a signing method as a back-up means for promoting total communication. I have seen this type of approach work amazingly well in severely deaf children. The encouragement given by understanding the signs always appears to stimulate their desire to use spoken words. Neither teacher, parent nor child ever use a sign alone, and they are inevitably accompanied by words, which now become more and more comprehensible because of the signs. This increasing comprehension leads to a greater desire to use expressive language. At first this is a sign plus a word, but as the combination is used more and more it is the sign that is gradually dropped, both by teacher, parent and child. The greater comprehension also stimulates cognition in general, so the child learns and can put signs together to express his thoughts and feelings, and as signs are always accompanied by words, he learns in this way to put words together. Short utterances, previously totally incomprehensible to the child, become meaningful because of the signs, and once again as he gains in confidence so the signs can be dropped.

It is important to use a sign language that provides grammar and syntax for the deaf child, for only in this way can his true ability be realized. It has been my misfortune to see quite a number of severely deaf children, that is not even the most profoundly deaf children, leaving school after 12 or so years of education, only able to lip-read the simplest of domestic instructions or use single words intelligibly (with perhaps a greater flow of words at home, but unintelligible to everyone except the mother and close siblings). They were able to 'read' but it was impossible to test their comprehension because their answers were unintelligible; often it appeared that their reading was purely mechanical. Number work did not exceed the mechanical areas because of their inability to understand the language of either problems or more difficult concepts. Such children were not unintelligent but nobody had provided them with the *means* of using their cognitive abilities and they were doomed to a life where, to support themselves, they had to take rather menial, mechanical jobs. Even when these jobs were done more than adequately, promotion was blocked because of their gross communication problems.

These young people certainly do 'retreat' to the deaf world. They frequently learn a simple signing system after leaving school, and then they can at least participate in the activities of special groups, clubs and even churches. This, of course, is why two deaf adults so often marry. In some cases this, of course, may be a good thing, supplying mutual support and understanding. There has even been some suggestion that the deaf offspring of two deaf parents tend to make better general progress than the deaf children of hearing parents. However, whereas no-one would give more than a passing thought to two non-genetic deaf persons marrying, it does seem rather tragic when two recessive genetic deaf adults are 'thrown' together because they have been virtually excluded from the normal hearing world through their lack of ability to communicate.

Gesture, of course, is the very best way of communicating affection; but gesture is normally accompanied by words – and the soft sound of 'I love you' can not really be replaced by the passing of written messages between the lovers. This, then, is just another example of what is denied to the deaf adult, who is sent out into the world unequipped to communicate as do most of his peers.

Obviously, then, there must be far more research into deaf education and money should be made available for this as a priority. Only recently have we realized that mental handicap should rate high in the competition for financial resources; now we should add the education of the deaf at the same level. Why, for example, is it not possible for *all* children to have the best radio-link equipment? Children in some areas are fortunate while others are not. Why is it not possible for *all* children to learn a signing system when this is deemed necessary? Again, some children are fortunate, while others are not.

The reader is referred to the work of Morris and Ives at the Royal Schools for the Deaf, Manchester, who amply illustrate the benefits of 'total communication' on the language development of deaf children[1].

SIGNING SYSTEMS

It is not the purpose of this book to describe the commonly used signing systems in any detail. The choice of a signing system is, in any case, probably more an educational than a medical problem. However we should be aware of what systems are available, with at least a very basic idea of their merits.

We have already commented above on the fact that all of us use gesture. Hearing people use gesture as a means of explaining, enlarging upon, emphasizing and even dramatizing their spoken words. How would the actor or the clown fare without his gesture? So gesture is a *natural* means of human communication. If, therefore, a person lacks one method of communication it seems wholly logical to develop another method. An analogy may be made with those people who lack sight, when their highly developed tactile sense enables them to use braille, and extend their cognitive abilities. In just such a way it seems to me that many hearing-impaired people are almost pleading to use gesture, controlled and systematized, as a means of extending their cognition. If this were not the case, why does the young deaf child 'sign' happily to his playmates in the playground, or the adolescents 'sign' to one another in their special clubs, at their coffee bars and discos? Yet time and time again this is ignored, or still in some cases frowned upon, by their teachers. Fortunately this has not always been the case and there are some schools where signing is available, and one gains the impression that the philosophy of 'total communication' is increasing.

There are many methods of non-oral communication which may be used, and probably each has a role to play for children with differing needs. On the other hand if many different types are in use then this diminishes the total number of people able to communicate with one another. It is probably true to say that a controlled study is necessary to find that system which best suits the *majority* of children with a severe hearing loss.

Whichever system is chosen there seems little doubt that it should be started at a very early age, so that the very young child grows up with speech, lip-reading and sign available and offered together. It is very interesting to see how the signs are dropped, both by child and parents, when the word, phrase, etc. is fully established, that is, spoken and understood orally.

In this chapter we can do little more than list the commonly used systems, but Appendix 2 gives the sources of greater information to those who wish to know more.

First, there is the *Paget–Gorman signing system*, developed by Lady Paget and Dr Pierre Gorman, an excellent system of communication which aims at introducing correct syntactical method into 'deaf communication'. In other words it is not 'signing shorthand' or merely 'telegrammatic speech' but a complete language. Children of normal intelligence usually learn it at a gratifyingly rapid rate, often somewhat faster than even the conscientious parents learning with them. It should, of course, be a family affair, and is of little value if limited to school. Both parents and other siblings should be strongly encouraged to learn the system, and many schools offer this facility themselves or else tell parents where it is available. The Paget-Gorman system is an excellent means of explaining more difficult concepts to the child who usually uses oral speech, having dropped signing for everyday language.

The second method, used much more commonly in the United States and Australia, is *cued speech*. One of the first aims of auditory training is to help the child to lip-read. But many sounds 'look' the same on the lips and the purpose of cued speech is to help the child distinguish the sounds by means of a manual sign which accompanies each phonetic part of the word. The system was devised in the United States by Orin Cornett, where great claims are made for the method. Its particular advantage is that it cannot be used without speech, and this aspect of it certainly prevents criticism from those people who maintain that 'signers never speak'. However, in the opinion of the writer, it is a harder system for families to learn. Each word used has to be broken down phonetically so that the correct sign can be used and parents and hearing siblings may find that they cannot do this quickly enough for the system to work efficiently. The evidence of success from the United States and Australia, however, does appear impressive, but this is probably the result of total family dedication combined with a total communication system.

The system, however, is of little use for children of below average intelligence and, as with all systems, the chances of success are highest when it can be commenced at a very early stage. At this stage the vocabulary used is small and all concerned get constant practice over a small number of words, which increases the probability of success with the harder and bigger vocabulary that must follow.

For children unable to use their hands competently, and who also have a hearing loss, neither of the above systems are suitable. For such children we can turn to *Bliss symbolic communication* or the *Makaton signing system*. The Bliss symbolic system, however, is mainly useful for children who have a reasonable degree of inner language and some verbal comprehension, but whose main difficulty lies in expressive speech. Therefore it applies to relatively few deaf children, where verbal comprehension is generally the main problem, but it may be useful for those cerebral palsied children whose hearing loss is a comparatively mild component of their total handicapping condition. It consists of sets of grouped symbols, commencing with 30 basic symbols and progressing to 400 symbols. The children indicate the appropriate symbols on a board, the signs being grouped appropriately according to their function, such as nouns, verbs, etc.

The Makaton system, however, was especially devised for children of very limited intelligence who also have a hearing loss (it is also, of course, very useful for severely retarded children with very little language resulting solely from their subnormality). It consists of a vocabulary which includes those words most commonly used and most essential for everyday living. The first stages are very basic, catering for children of very limited ability. But further stages proceed to more advanced vocabulary and then on to more complex language concepts. The child can be taken as far as his abilities allow. Unlike the Paget–Gorman system it is not intended to convey the syntactical ideas of normal language. It is said, in fact, that this system has 'grown' out of the signs which the deaf commonly use among themselves, and which we have already mentioned above in this book. Perhaps we may say that it is the logical conclusion of 'playground signing'. But if it can be combined with finger-spelling, lip-reading and some speech, in more able children, then it becomes possible to introduce some grammatical form. In addition the signs used in this system do not carry strict rules for their performance, so once again the much less able child or the child with poorer manual competence can benefit very greatly from its use. The enormous value of this system, then, is its flexibility.

We have left until last, the *British signing system*. Several useful books have been written about this, some in a very simple and easily understood way[2,3]. This signing system is best used together with finger spelling. The signs are made mainly by the hands, but the hands are also used in relation to the head and body. For example the sign for *I* consists of the very natural gesture in which the index finger of the right hand points towards oneself. Similarly the sign for *my* or *mine* is similar to the sign for *I* except that the fist is closed to indicate that something is possessed. Critics would say that this is purely pantomime and leaves out many of the important little words, thus producing telegrammatic speech. But when one remembers the limitation in amount of expressive speech and verbal comprehension in so many deaf school leavers then surely it is better to systematize the signs that they use to one another, so that parents, friends, social workers and even some sympathetic employers may take the trouble to learn this simple signing system and thus increase the link between the adolescent and his new environment. This is particularly vital when the young person leaves a sheltered school life to take up a job in a hearing world.

Whatever form of signing is used, it should *never* be used without speech; signing should always play its part in *total communication*. The deaf person needs good amplification, good auditory, speech and language training plus a suitable signing system whenever oral speech alone does not allow him to fulfil his complete potential. The addition of a signing system, then, used as described above, *never* hinders the production of oral speech. On the other hand by the encouragement induced by success in communication, the child is spurred on to greater attempts in all kinds of communication, including speech.

References

1. Morris, T. (1978). *The Effect of Total Communication on the Language Development of Two Groups of Deaf Children.* (Manchester: The Rycroft Centre, Royal School for the Deaf)

2. Jones, H. and Willis, L. (1972). *Talking Hands: an Introduction to Communicating with People who are Deaf.* (London: Stanley Paul) [Based on a series of programmes on Tyne-Tees Television. This book may be borrowed from the library at the RNID.]

3. Cormat, P.T. (1971). *Ten Graded Exercises in Manual Communication for Learners.* (Published by the author) [This book can be bought from the British Deaf Association, 38 Victoria Place, Carlisle, or borrowed from the RNID library.]

Chapter 15

PROBLEMS OF THE MIDDLE EAR

The anatomy of the middle ear has already been described in Chapter 4, together with its role in the passage of sound from its source to the nerve endings in the inner ear.

We have also seen that problems in the middle ear, giving rise to what is known, for obvious reasons, as *conductive deafness*, produce audiograms in which the air conduction indicates the level of the problem while the bone conduction remains normal. In other words the passage of sound straight into the temporal bone bypasses the lesion in the middle ear passing straight to the inner ear. Thus the audiogram shows what is known as an 'air–bone gap', characteristic of a conductive hearing loss. In sensorineural hearing loss it does not matter at all where the sound enters, if the all-important cochlea is damaged. However, it is important to remember at this point that children with a sensorineural hearing loss are certainly not immune to factors such as recurrent upper respiratory tract infections, which cause chronic secretory otitis media or 'glue ear', so they may get a conductive element added to the sensorineural loss. In such cases an air–bone gap can often be seen, and it is important to treat the conductive element vigorously and thus perhaps improve the impaired hearing by anything from 5 to around 20 dB, especially in the lower frequencies. The child who needs to wear a hearing aid is

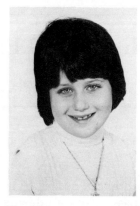

Fig 41a

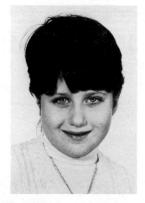

Fig 41b

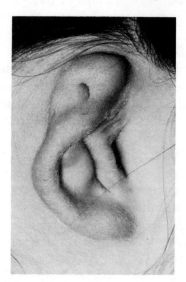

Fig 41c

Figure 41 (a) Apparently normal little girl. (b) Note the difference between right and left ears. (c) Close-up of right ear; external auditory meatus is closed; hearing is normal on the left side. There is *no family history* of a similar deformity

usually very pleased by this improvement and parents often comment on the marked difference in the child's general responsiveness. To a child with a very serious hearing loss these few decibels are precious.

The common lesions found in the middle ear may be divided into two main types, the congenital type and the infective type.

CONGENITAL MIDDLE EAR LESIONS

We have already remarked in Chapter 11 on some of the congenital forms, such as otosclerosis. This, however, is inherited in a dominant form and there are many children who have isolated congenital lesions without any traceable family history. Such children may show abnormalities of the malleus, or of the joints between the ossicles, and, very commonly, of the stapes. The footplate of the stapes may not be in the oval window, or the oval window itself may be abnormal in shape or position, or may be absent. In some children such lesions are associated with cleft palate or congenital lesions in other systems. Some of them merely have asymmetric or unusual facies, which seems to give a clue to the presence of abnormalities in the middle ear. Sometimes the symptoms and signs appear to be those of 'glue ear' but myringotomy yields no 'glue', while perhaps a later tympanotomy shows the abnormality of the ossicles and other middle ear structures. In some cases the surgeon can refashion the ossicles, or replace them so that they articulate. Artificial 'joints' may be made and even the membrane can be refashioned, to cover the oval window if this should prove to be part of the problem.

INFECTIVE MIDDLE EAR LESIONS

The infective causes of conductive hearing loss are by far the most common and widespread. The reason for this has already been indicated in the easy access of organisms from the nose, throat and nasopharynx to the middle ear through the eustachian tube or pharyngotympanic tube. Therefore the child who has recurrent upper respiratory tract infections (and here we must include that troublesome phenomenon, the 'catarrhal child' who is a problem to himself, to his family and to his doctor) also falls easily prey to infections of the middle ear. This type of child commonly also has enlarged adenoids, which act as a block to the eustachian tube.

The child complains of pain or discomfort in the ear, the doctor finds a typically inflamed eardrum and prescribes an antibiotic. The mucous membrane of the middle ear, and the eustachian tube, secretes a thin inflammatory fluid, which is really an exacerbation of the normal mucus secreted by the mucous membrane lining of the middle ear in its healthy state. In many cases the administration of an *adequate* course of antibiotic, which is given regularly to the patient and not discarded as soon as the earache ceases, does two important things. First it prevents the secretory discharge from being purulent, with subsequent rupture of the drum, as already described in Chapter 4, and secondly it clears up the excessive mucoid discharge which has already occurred, so that the eustachian tube can reopen and air can again pass into the middle ear. However, all too often, the family cease giving the antibiotic when the symptoms subside. In these cases, although no purulent discharge is formed, the mucoid discharge is not absorbed and remains in the middle ear as a sterile effusion. When the child gets its next upper respiratory tract infection, even possibly without earache, the performance is repeated and finally the ear becomes filled with the mucoid discharge which tends to thicken, becoming almost gelatinous in nature. In addition, because of the repeated infectious processes, the eustachian tube similarly becomes completely blocked, so that instead of a eustachian tube and middle ear cleft being filled with air, both structures

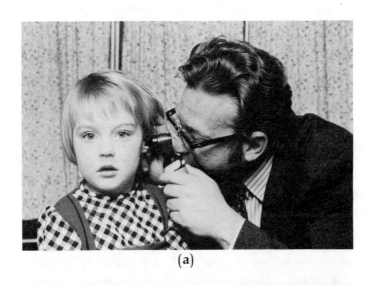

(a)

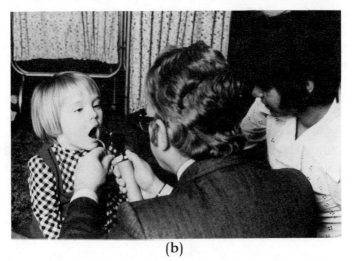

(b)

Figure 42   Examining (a) the tympanic membrane; (b) the
tonsils and palate

are filled with this thick, viscous, mucoid material, which cannot be absorbed or drain away. This is the typical picture of 'glue ear', and it is easy for the reader to see how the term arises.

The clinical picture of the tympanic membrane in glue ear or, as we should properly call it, *chronic secretory (or serous) otitis media*, is easy to recognize, with practice (although even the best clinicians can sometimes be mistaken). The drum is retracted, because of the negative pressure created within the middle ear by the closure of the eustachian tube. The landmarks normally seen on the drum (that is, the handle of the malleus with its short lateral process at the upper end, and the light reflex usually made by a reflection of the light cast by the examiner's instrument on the drum in this area – see Figure 5) are often missing. The light reflex may be seen but may be very dull. The colour of the whole membrane may be abnormal; it is often described as 'bluish' but, on the other hand, it is often mildly inflamed, being generally pink in appearance and showing individual dilated vessels. The commonest features at the commencement of this condition are the retraction of the drum and the general dullness of its appearance. In contrast a healthy tympanic membrane looks almost shiny grey in colour, with a well-defined hammer handle and a bright light reflex.

As may be expected the presence of the thick mucoid material in the middle ear interferes with its normal function. None of the structures in the middle ear can move normally in response to sound stimuli and a hearing loss of anything up to 40 dB, in the worst cases, may result. The hearing loss tends to be worse in the low frequencies, particularly at 500 Hz, and hearing at 2 kHz and 4 kHz *may* be normal. Bone conduction shows normal hearing.

The final proof, for the clinician who has seen a suspicious tympanic membrane and found a hearing loss as described above, is the result of tympanometry, using an acoustic impedance bridge (Figure 43). The modern tympanometer is now so simple to operate that a probe is placed in the child's

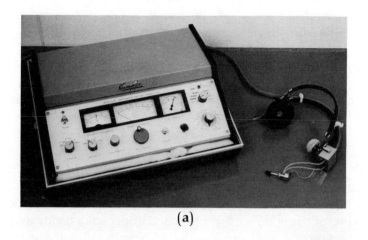

(a)

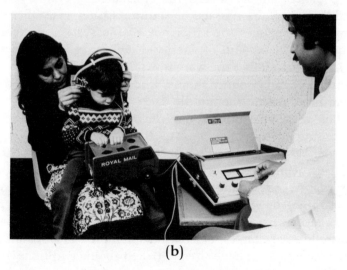

(b)

Figure 43 (a) The acoustic impedance bridge used for tympanometry and the measurement of stapedial reflexes. (b) Use of the bridge on a rather unwilling patient, but the apparatus was successfully held in place

ear, a button is pressed, and a graph indicating the pressure in the middle ear is printed out in a matter of seconds. Because of the speed of the test it is possible to use the machine with babies, which is particularly helpful.

TYMPANOMETRY

The pressure in the middle ear, as mentioned above, is virtually the same as external air pressure, provided that the eustachian tube is open and healthy. If for any reason there is a difference in pressure between the outer and middle ears this reduces the mobility, or what we may also call 'the compliance' of the tympanic membrane.

Conversely we can say 'the impedance' of the whole system of the middle ear is increased under such conditions. 'Impedance' simply means the resistance offered by the middle ear to the passage of sound. Greater resistance to movement reduces the efficiency of the system and consequently the amount of energy reaching the cochlea.

Investigation into the way in which the middle ear reacts to an incoming sound should lead to information about conditions within the middle ear.

The resistance offered by the middle ear also varies according to the frequency of the sound used. At high frequencies the resistance is mainly due to the mass of the ossicles. On the other hand, at low frequencies, the impedance or resistance is principally due to the stiffness of the supporting structures and the connecting ligaments. In this chapter, we are, of course, concerned with conditions in the middle ear that, for one reason or another, cause changes in its stiffness. We have already talked about conditions that vary from one end of the 'resistance spectrum' to the other – otosclerosis, for example, in which healthy bone is replaced by immature spongy bone which encroaches on to the periphery of the oval window and finally involves the whole base plate of the stapes, thus causing the junction of the stapes and the membrane covering the oval window to be totally immobile. On the other hand congenital abnormalities of the middle ear, and abnormal ossicles, or abnormalities of the ossicular joints, may lead to *ossicular discontinuity*. This may mean that the weak link in the chain causes the tympanic membrane to become unusually mobile, in other words its impedance is decreased. As we are mainly concerned with changes of stiffness, and this particularly applies to the commonest condition discussed, 'glue ear', we use a low frequency sound for testing.

Also, in testing, we do not in fact measure impedance, but its inverse, 'compliance' or the mobility of the middle ear.

We have already stated that any difference in pressure between the outer and middle ear reduces the compliance of the tympanic membrane and we can now expand this a little by stating that a pressure differential of $\frac{1}{2}\%$ (0.5%) is enough to halve the compliance of the tympanic membrane. With a pressure differential of approximately 2% the membrane becomes effectively rigid and compliance reaches a minimum.

Therefore, if an excess pressure of 2% is artificially applied in the external canal over a normal middle ear, compliance becomes minimal (this can be achieved by means of an air pump incorporated in the apparatus). As the pressure differential is reduced the compliance rises and there is a sharp peak at the point where the pressure in the external canal is exactly equal to that in the middle ear. In the normal ear this happens at atmospheric pressure. As the pressure in the external canal is reduced the compliance again falls to a minimal value, where there is approximately 2% difference between the pressures inside and outside the middle ear. In this way, by finding the external canal pressure at which the compliance of the middle ear system is maximal, the pressure inside the middle ear can be measured, and a graph may be plotted.

In cases where there is eustachian malfunction, with

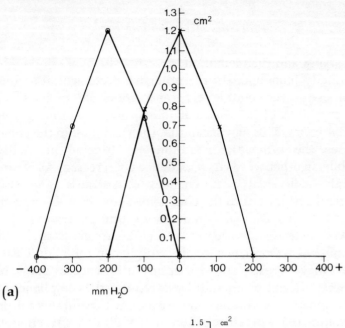

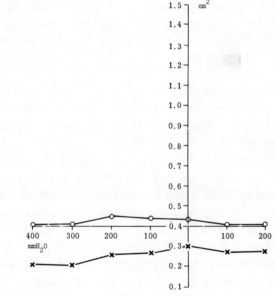

Figure 44 (a) × Graph illustrating normal impedance curve (left ear); ○ graph illustrating eustachian catarrh (right ear). (b) Graph illustrating 'flat' result in impedance test in glue ear: ○ right ear, × left ear

closure of the tube as described in cases of infection of the middle ear, there is negative pressure in the middle ear, with retraction of the drum, and the peak of compliance occurs at a negative pressure, such as -100 or -200 mmH$_2$O.

If, however, there is a collection of thick mucoid material in the middle ear, then the changes of pressure in the external canal have no effect at all, as the middle ear structures have been effectively prevented from moving by the products of repeated infection. Thus a flat curve is produced (see Figures 44(a) and (b)).

The same piece of apparatus can also measure the *stapedial reflex*. It was stated in Chapter 4 that the function of the stapedius and tensor tympani muscles is probably to protect the structures of the middle ear at very loud sound intensities, that is at around 70 dB above the threshold of hearing of the individual. Thus, normally the stapedius contraction can be measured at 90 dB, where 20 dB is taken as the limit of normal hearing. Machines vary in the frequencies at which the stapedial reflex is measured. The modern machine already mentioned measures only at 90 dB at 1 kHz. Other machines, less fully automated, have the advantage of measuring at 500 Hz, and 1 kHz, 2 kHz, and 3 kHz. They also measure at 90 dB, 100 dB, 110 dB and 120 dB. The latter is useful as it is another method of checking hearing loss in young children and is fully objective. Children with severe sensorineural hearing loss do not, of course, show any stapedial reflex. Neither can it be registered in children whose middle ears are full of 'glue'.

TREATMENT OF INFECTIVE CONDITIONS OF THE MIDDLE EAR

As mentioned above acute otitis media is treated promptly with antibiotic and it should be stressed to the parents that treatment should *not* be stopped because symptoms have subsided. Some parents often store the antibiotic, using it again without medical advice, and in a similar inadequate fashion, when the child next complains of discomfort in the ear. By doing this strains of organisms are produced immune to the effects of varying antibiotics. The dose and length of course, therefore, should be very clearly stated to the parents and they should be advised to throw away any remains at the end of the bottle after completing the course conscientiously; reasons for this should be explained wherever possible and practicable. The habit of 'leaving out a prescription' for an unseen patient is a very poor medical practice, even when the family is well known to the doctor.

The treatment of chronic secretory otitis media or glue ear is very important indeed, because of the effect on hearing. We have mentioned above the figure of 5 % of children who at or around the age of $4\frac{1}{2}$ to 5 years, that is at school entry age, show a conductive hearing loss which has already interfered with their acquisition of speech at the normal age. Much important and interesting research has been done on the subject by Hamilton and Owrid.[1] Without treatment these children go on to show difficulties in learning to read at the normal age. It is obvious that the diagnosis of small conductive hearing losses in very young children is *very important*.

In fact the careful observer can find many examples of young babies whose hearing tests are not completely satisfactory, although they do not show any gross loss suggestive of a sensorineural loss. It may be found, for instance, that normal hearing responses are not obtained to the usual tests at the accurate screening levels described, although they are obtained if the sound stimuli are increased to around 50 dB. Examination of the tympanic membranes may well show them to be dull and somewhat retracted, thus indicating that the very short eustachian tubes in the infant are not functioning optimally. In such cases the mother should be asked to use a rather raised voice with very meaningful words when talking to the infant, as she works or particularly when she is feeding, bathing, or dressing him. When playing with him she should turn the baby round on her knee so that he can also *see* her lips moving, as she uses her slightly raised voice. Such an infant should be kept under careful supervision to make sure that the condition subsides. On the whole I do not favour using antihistamines (see below) in babies under about 18 months of age, but they may be useful in particular cases when the condition seems recurrent or obstinate at this very young age.

The use of antihistamines is the second line of treatment. There is a large school of thought that considers the secretions found in the eustachian tube and the middle ear to be the response to an allergic condition, in addition to an infection. Thus the use of antihistamines would be quite logical, and in the acute phase perhaps the combination of antibiotic plus antihistamine would be more effective in preventing the subsequent onset of the chronic phase.

Certainly in children where there is no previous history of ear symptoms, where recurrent upper respiratory tract infections are *not* the rule, and in very young children, there seems to be a very definite indication for the treatment of chronic secretory otitis media with a relatively long course of antihistamines, particularly where there is a personal or family history of other allergic conditions. It is also useful in chronic cases who have perhaps had two or three sets of grommets inserted, and whose tympanic membranes show the results of repeated surgery and obviously would not benefit from further interference. The length of course usually recommended initially is about 6 weeks, but this can be extended.

There are many different proprietary brands of anti-histamine and the one chosen is probably largely a matter of a doctor's individual preference. But as they often tend to make children sleepy it is advisable to commence with a single dose at bedtime for a day or so, before gradually increasing the dose to twice and then thrice daily, according to the age of the child. In addition, some antihistamines make a child bad-tempered and markedly irritable. If this does not wear off within a day or so as the child becomes accustomed to the drug, then it should be changed to a different proprietary brand. The results of an antihistamine course vary widely. Some parents report no difference in symptoms, while others say that a nasal discharge has cleared and that the hearing has somewhat improved. This, of course, can be checked by clinical tests and by audiometry and impedance where practicable.

Finally there is the surgical treatment of the condition by means of myringotomy, sucking out the contents of the middle ear and eustachian tube, and the insertion of a small plastic tube or grommet which has a little flange at each end to stop it coming out of the tympanic membrane. It remains in place, coming through the tympanic membrane, for a very varying length of time, anything from 6 weeks to 6 months. As the tympanic membrane heals it pushes the grommet out into the external auditory canal and it usually disappears without patient or parent being aware of this. Sometimes if it is lying in the external auditory canal, having finished its useful life, the ENT surgeon removes it very simply, through a speculum. (*Note*: This is *not* a job for an amateur, and the grommet does no harm if left lying in the external canal.)

What is the real purpose of the grommet? The thick mucoid material would not drain out of it, so must be *actively* sucked out of the middle ear, etc. before the grommet is inserted. But the all-important purpose of the grommet is to let air into the middle ear again. As the healthy middle ear is one that is filled with air, the presence of the grommet also allows the middle ear to function again.

The effect of the insertion of grommets into the middle ear is usually quite spectacular as regards the improvement in hearing. Within the matter of a week or so – or even a day or so – parents comment on this improvement. In some cases

this improvement is sustained for long periods, but unfortunately there is a marked tendency for the condition to
recur until around 6 or 7 years, when it becomes much less
common. By this age most children have developed an
immunity to the common organisms and the increasing
length and width of the eustachian tube also helps to keep
the middle ear aerated.

In the meantime, unfortunately it is often necessary to
insert grommets on more than one occasion. An interesting
piece of research[2] has shown that the final result in the
hearing of a group of children treated by myringotomies and
grommets whenever necessary, was the same as a group of
children treated purely conservatively, when both groups
reached the age of 6 to 7 years. This has been advanced as an
argument to 'prove' that surgical treatment is unnecessary
interference, with the ever-present risks of anaesthesia,
however small these are. But this argument fails to take into
consideration the harm done by perhaps 6 years of recurrent
hearing loss, at a vital time in the child's development of
language and also, more important, when the child starts
school. Judicious treatment with grommets gives the young
child long periods of normal or very nearly normal hearing
when speech therapists can work hard to help the child who
is already retarded in his speech development. The operation for insertion of grommets can be done as a 'day' case.
But if adenoidectomy is necessary, as it often is, then 2 to 3
days in hospital is required.

Children who are sufficiently unfortunate to develop
spontaneous perforations of the tympanic membrane, with
purulent discharge, or mucopurulent discharge, should be
given vigorous antibiotic treatment, and in many cases if the
condition is treated promptly the perforation heals, although some diminution of hearing may remain due to the
scarring, thickening and adhesions. If the condition is
neglected by parents, who are not unduly worried because
the child is not crying with pain, the perforation may

become chronic. Discharge may occur on and off, with long periods of dry ear. The amount of hearing loss varies but is not very great, especially when one considers the size of some of these perforations. (The reader must *always* remember, however, that even a *small* hearing loss can interfere with language, education, emotional and social development, so that it should not automatically be lightly dismissed.) There is no doubt that this type of chronic perforation is best treated surgically, by myringoplasty. In this operation the surgeon creates a new tympanic membrane by grafting various materials into the area of the old tympanic membrane which has been thoroughly cleaned by removal of all old infective material. The material used for the graft has varied from skin (which proved unsuccessful after a time, when the skin broke down and perished), to connective tissue available from the temporal fascia, a dura homograft and a total replacement with the ossicles attached, that is, a whole tympanic membrane obtained from a cadaver used to replace the unhealthy parts of the patient's own middle ear. The commonest methods now in use are the temporal fascia and dura homografts.

It was finally realized that often attention to the tympanic membrane alone was insufficient, and some restoration of the connection between the drum and the oval window had to be insured, with adequate working of the eustachian tube. Thus, a myringoplasty could become an involved piece of plastic surgery in cases where the ossicles and eustachian tube were also chronically diseased, and could now be more accurately called a tympanoplasty. However such operations now are usually very successful, and greatly to be recommended, with varying degrees of increase in the hearing, and the considerable advantage of a 'dry' ear.

We should not leave the question of middle ear conditions without mentioning *cholesteatoma*. In this, the now familiar story of recurrent upper respiratory tract infections causes infection of the adenoids, which is also very common. These normally small pads of lymphoid tissue swell, as a reaction to the infections, thus causing mouth-breathing, snoring, and more importantly obstruction of the openings of the eustachian tubes. (It is because of these important signs and symptoms that in such children the operation of myring-otomy with insertion of grommets is often accompanied by adenoidectomy.) Where this is neglected there is chronic obstruction of the eustachian tube and chronic lack of middle ear aeration, causing a chronic state of negative pressure in the middle ear. This, as we have stated, causes retraction of the drum which is easily seen on auroscopic examination. At the same time, in the cases under discussion, there is a slow and undiscovered disturbance in the normal migration of the keratin shed by the outermost layer of the tympanic membrane.

Normally the cells on this surface move from the centre of the tympanic membrane towards the periphery and are finally 'shed' and move out of the meatus. But in these particular children the keratin moves to fill up the pocket which is made by the drum as it retracts. Eventually the weakest part of the retracted drum gives way and the keratin deposit enters the middle ear through the perfor-ation. As time goes by more and more keratin enters and is laid down around the original deposit. This extraordinary process continues until the abnormal deposit threatens to occupy the whole of the middle ear and surrounding areas, for, although as would be expected a cholesteatoma is soft in consistency it can actually invade bone and cause havoc not only in the middle ear but also in the surrounding areas. The whole process is very insidious, until finally a cold which is accompanied by a foul-smelling discharge from the ears may bring the whole situation to light. Fortunately this condition has become much rarer in children now and is usually seen in those from Third World countries where medical help is not so easily available. The writer has a good example of this now attending her clinic, a 16-year-old boy recently arrived in the United Kingdom from a very remote part of Bangladesh. (We have even had considerable difficulty in finding adults from his own country who could understand his own particular dialect.)

When such a condition is encountered it obviously requires a vigorous combined medical and surgical attack. The amount of hearing loss accompanying this condition obviously depends on the extent of the lesion and the structures that have been invaded.

Lastly we must mention accidental injury to the middle ear, and also remember that occasionally this tragically forms part of the *non*-accidental injuries inflicted on children. It is usually associated with fracture of the base of the skull, in which bleeding from the ear can almost be a diagnostic symptom. The ossicle most commonly affected is the incus as it is least well supplied with ligaments. Obviously the extent of the injury and the question of whether the oval window is involved determines the extent of the conductive deafness or the presence of sensorineural deafness after such an accident. Some of the children arriving from Vietnam, at the time of the war there, showed in the middle ear the results of blast from bombs or guns. The writer has a small patient, now happily settled in Kent, and using good colloquial English, whose war injury affecting the middle ear was recently tidied up by surgery and followed by a tympanoplasty. One of his main ambitions was to swim, with his new family, and this is now possible. His hearing on the injured side showed a marked conductive loss, before treatment, but as his other ear was normal this, together with understanding parents and teachers, compensated to a very large degree.

References

1. Hamilton, P. and Owrid, H.L. (1974). *Br. J. Audiol.*, **8**

(Feb.)

2. Brown, M.J.K.M., Richard, S.H. and Ambegaskar, A.G. (1978). Grommets and glue ear: a five-year follow-up of a controlled trial. *J. R. Soc. Med.*, **71**, 5

Chapter 16

DEAFNESS ASSOCIATED WITH MENTAL HANDICAP

First of all we must reiterate that the ability of a deaf child *must* be assessed by suitable means, that is, by performance tests that do not rely on any verbal instructions or answers. This has been mentioned already but I do not apologize for stressing it as the most surprising reports are sometimes submitted with a child sent for review of a hearing loss. As the educational psychologist is responsible for a child's school placement it is obviously essential that he or she is aware of a hearing loss, be it large or small, together with all its implications. For example the question of whether a child is placed in a partially-hearing unit or a school for the severely mentally handicapped (ESN(s) school) is of crucial importance and depends very largely on the psychologist's final recommendation.

However, there is no doubt at all that mental handicap of varying degrees is commonly associated with hearing loss. If items in Table 3, illustrating causes of hearing loss and mental subnormality, are compared the reasons for this will be immediately obvious.

Causes at conception in both cases contain conditions caused by autosomal dominant genes, by autosomal recessive genes and X-linked genes.

The branchial arch syndromes, for example, are inherited in a dominant manner. Patients with syndromes such as

Table 3 Aetiology of mental subnormality

Causes before or at conception	Prenatal causes	Causes at or around birth	Causes after birth
1. Genetic, due to genes of small effect (clinically undifferentiated)	1. Physical, such as irradiation	1. Prematurity*	1. Infections such as meningitis, encephalitis* (measles, etc.)
2. Genetic, due to genes of large effect	2. *Chemical, such as thalidomide	2. Low birth-weight*	2. Infantile spasms
Dominant	3. *Biological, such as; infections in pregnancy – rubella; cytomegalovirus; congenital toxoplasmosis; syphilis	3. Obstetric problems, such as APH prolapsed cord (anoxic problems)*	3. Lead poisoning
Tuberose sclerosis	4. Unknown causes, such as Sturge–Weber syndrome; Rubinstein–Taybi syndrome; Cornelia de Lange syndrome (Amsterdam dwarf)	4. Hyaline membrane disease (respiratory distress syndrome)*	
Neurofibromatosis (Von Recklinghausen's disease)		5. Hypoglycaemia	
*Waardenburg's syndrome		6. Hyperbilirubinaemia*	
*Acrocephaly			
Syndromes with myotonia and retardation			
Recessive			
Phenylketonuria			
Homocystinuria			
Maple syrup disease			
Hepatolenticular degeneration (Wilson's disease)			
Galactosaemia			
Lipidoses (Tay–Sachs disease)			
Leukodystrophies			
Mucopolysaccharidoses (Hurler's syndrome)			
*(Hunter's syndrome) (X)			

3. Primary chromosomal abnormalities

   Downs syndrome (47)*
   Cri-du-Chat (deletion short arm 5)
   Patau's syndrome (extra in pair 13–15)*
   Edwards' syndrome (extra in pair 18)
   Klinefelter's syndrome (XXY)
   XYY syndrome
   Turner's syndrome (XO)*

4. *Deafness associated with multiple congenital deformities**

   Craniofacial dysostosis (Crouzon's disease) (D)
   Mandibulofacial dysostosis (Treacher–Collins) (D)
   Pierre Robin syndrome (D)
   Otopalatodigital syndrome (D)
   Oculoauriculovertebral dysplasia (D)
   Lawrence–Moon–Biedl–Bardet syndrome (R)

Key: *Indicates the possibility of deafness occurring with this condition; (D) = dominant; (R) = Recessive; (X) = X-linked.

205

Treacher–Collins (see pages 123–4) often show normal intelligence but this is by no means invariable, and the writer has already referred to the case with which she is best acquainted, where the boy is severely mentally handicapped. Similarly, craniofacial dysostosis (Crouzon's disease) is often associated with both conductive hearing loss and mental subnormality. Oculoauriculovertebral dysplasia in which ocular abnormalities may be associated with facial asymmetry, macrostomia, scoliosis and auricular appendages, can be similarly associated with both conductive hearing loss and varying degrees of mental handicap.

It should be noted that patients with Waardenburg's syndrome (see page 121), although this appears in the table, usually have normal intelligence.

Lawrence–Moon–Biedl–Bardet syndrome (see page 117), although a comparatively rare condition, is seen from time to time in hospital practice and is an example found in the table. This is inherited in a recessive manner, is quite often associated with deafness, and is yet another condition in which the degree of intelligence is very variable.

The outstanding example of an X-linked inherited condition, in which both mental subnormality and deafness are found together is Hunter's syndrome (see Chapter 11).

The above are only a very few examples of a great many conditions, many of them rare, which are inherited in one way or another and in which mental retardation goes hand in hand with hearing loss. The important point to be made is that where several cases of mental subnormality are found within a family it is extremely important to do careful hearing tests. (Note also the comments on hearing tests of the mentally subnormal in Chapter 17).

Deafness is also found quite frequently in conditions due to chromosomal abnormalities. The important condition to remember here, since cases are reasonably frequent, is Down's syndrome or mongolism. Very young children with Down's syndrome frequently show a definite conductive hearing loss. This is due to their tendency to frequent upper respiratory tract infections and general 'snuffliness' which is such an obvious feature of their general condition; they are specially prone to chronic secretory otitis media (see Chapter 15). At the right age they can often be helped by the insertion of grommets. If another condition, such as a congenital heart lesion, makes an anaesthetic for this insertion undesirable, then they can be taught to use hearing aids quite successfully. The writer has had several such children attending her clinic who use hearing aids with considerable benefit to their slow acquisition of some language.

Other much rarer chromosomal abnormalities are sometimes associated with deafness. An extra chromosome in pairs 13–15 (Patou's syndrome), and an extra chromosome in pair 18 (Edwards' syndrome) are examples. We have also seen an example of the Cri-du-Chat syndrome (deletion of the short arm of 5) and at least two other cases with varying deletions, and very definite sensorineural hearing loss. Turner's syndrome (XO) can also show a hearing loss.

In view of the above examples once again we may say that all children with known or suspected chromosomal abnormalities should have a very careful hearing test.

The causes of both mental subnormality and deafness occurring in pregnancy, are remarkably similar, as will again be seen from the table. This is hardly surprising as the biggest group is that caused by infections in pregnancy, the biggest culprit of all being rubella, which has already been discussed at some length (Chapter 12). Cytomegalovirus (CMV) and toxoplasmosis are known though rarer causes of mental subnormality with deafness. In all these cases the organism, especially when it infects early in pregnancy, harms many developing areas of the tiny fetus. Thus it should be no surprise, in the absence of abortion, to find many parts of the infant affected by what can only be described as a catastrophe.

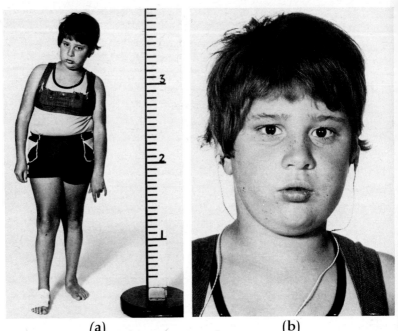

(a)   (b)

Figure 45   (a) and (b) Chromosomal abnormality; transloca-
tion of chromosome 17, showing both severe deafness and
severe mental handicap

Syphilis should be included in this group, but thanks to
the modern routine testing of antenatal patients, together
with more adequate treatment of the disease, one is unlikely
to find such a case in a busy clinic.

The possible effect of drugs in pregnancy has been
highlighted by the thalidomide tragedies. Thalidomide
itself, however, did not seem a major cause of mental
handicap. In fact the common 'picture' of thalidomide
children has been that of children of normal, even above
average, intelligence, learning to cope with their gross
physical abnormalities; these have sometimes included
abnormalities of the ears, but again this has not been a
common picture.

As we have already discussed, premature infants and low birth-weight infants are especially liable to hearing loss and are also more prone to mental subnormality. Premature infants have the better prognosis especially when treated in specialized intensive care units. Low birth-weight infants when carefully monitored antenatally and induced prematurely at the crucial moment, or delivered by caesarean section, have a better prognosis if treated in the intensive care unit rather than staying *in utero*, with the hazard of poor nourishment from the placenta. In both cases the addition of anoxia from any other cause greatly increases the risk of both mental subnormality and hearing loss.

Anoxia from any of the causes that have already been discussed is a common cause of subnormality, although as obstetric practice improves the number of unhappy sequelae decreases. However, the standard of obstetric practice varies and the Spastics Society rightly campaigns vigorously for an improvement in obstetric care at all stages. Subnormality caused by lack of vital oxygen supply *in utero* at the time of or shortly after birth (as in hyaline membrane disease) is commonly accompanied by symptoms caused by the effect of the anoxia on specific areas. Thus not only deafness, due to haemorrhage into the inner ear, but conditions such as cerebral palsy, epilepsy, etc., may all be present together. Cerebral palsy in fact is very commonly accompanied by hearing loss.

In the postnatal period hyperbilirubinaemia is an extremely dangerous condition for the infant unless diagnosed and treated promptly (see Chapter 12). The kernicterus which causes deafness by toxic damage to the cochlear nuclei etc. (see Chapter 12) also commonly causes athetoid cerebral palsy as well as mental subnormality. The risk of damage is much greater in premature infants or those of low birth-weight, when much lower levels of the serum bilirubin may prove dangerous. Also in such infants 'physiological' jaundice rather than that caused by blood

incompatibilities may give rise to the raised serum bilirubin
levels and the danger of athetoid cerebral palsy with mental
subnormality and hearing loss.

Fortunately this problem is becoming much rarer for two
reasons. First the treatment of infants showing a raised
serum bilirubin has improved enormously (see Chapter 12)
and secondly the prophylactic treatment of those women at
risk after the birth of their first baby because of blood
incompatibilities has become almost routine (see Chapter
12).

Although the prompt diagnosis and much more effective
treatment of meningitis, with a range of antibiotics that deal
very efficiently with most of the common organisms
involved, is an example where the incidence of mental
subnormality as a sequel has decreased, the incidence of
hearing loss remains depressingly high at around 5%.
Presumably the close anatomical relationship between the
inner ear, bathed in its perilymph, which drains into the
cerebrospinal fluid is the reason for this.

The rare but dangerous complication of measles (measles
encephalitis) may similarly result both in very severe mental
retardation, and occasionally in addition, in hearing loss.

The examples quoted are meant to help the reader
appreciate that the causes of both mental subnormality and
hearing loss 'overlap' to a very considerable degree. Thus it
would seem obvious that hearing loss should be sought very
vigorously among those children who show signs of general
retardation. Unhappily this has not been true until fairly
recently and, even now, there must be large numbers of
adults in subnormality hospitals who also have an undiagnosed – and certainly untreated – hearing loss, which of
course, increases their inability to communicate and to
learn, whereas if their hearing loss is discovered and treated
their prognosis may be altered quite startlingly. A young
mentally subnormal adult, turned in upon himself by a
severe hearing loss, may alter very markedly with the gentle

introduction of a simple sign language, such as the Makaton system (page 179), together with the individual interest and help provided for him by an interested and enthusiastic speech therapist. No miracles can be expected here but the quality of life may be distinctly improved by the diagnosis and treatment of a hearing loss in the young or young–middle-aged mentally subnormal patient.

Another myth that must be dispelled is that such patients cannot use a hearing aid. Very young handicapped patients may reject their aids vigorously, but we have been able to show that by very slow, patient, conditioning techniques, with suitable reward systems, even the most difficult children can be persuaded to use amplification.* Let me add at once that this depends entirely upon the quality of the staff who are using these techniques, and I have often had cause to be very thankful for the skill, patience and love shown towards their little patients, who for so long appeared so unrewarding.

We must also be entirely realistic in what we hope to achieve by the use of both amplification and a signing system in patients who demonstrate two such major handicaps together. In the case of amplification I hope that we may be able to give the patient some pleasure, some increased awareness of his or her environment and, hopefully, an alerting mechanism for some dangers. In the case of a child it is extremely useful (and not entirely negative) if the child can hear and comprehend a very loudly spoken 'NO', which may quite often prevent an accident. Another example is the usefulness of such a patient being able to *hear* traffic and to be taught the connections between the noise and the danger.

In patients with more ability, provided they are caught

---

* I would like to pay tribute to the staff at Hilda Lewis House, Bethlem Royal Hospital, who have shown by their enthusiastic and patient work that this can be done.

young enough, for example, young patients who are 'high grade' mongols, both their comprehension of speech and expressive language can certainly be increased. For those with less ability their pleasure in music and interesting sounds can often be increased. In addition they may be able to acquire at least a little communication through a simple signing system.

There are still some cases who appear to be of lesser ability than is their true potential because of an undiagnosed hearing loss. This may be particularly so in cases of athetoid cerebral palsy, where hearing should be carefully supervised. I have already mentioned (page 129) a little girl with Hurler's syndrome, whose undiagnosed hearing loss certainly confused the picture of her true intelligence.

I can well remember those days when no attempt was made to measure the hearing or vision of the severely mentally handicapped. The attitude, then, was 'What does it matter?' I hope the answer to this question is now more than clear and that every effort, using both subjective and objective tests, should be made, to get a true picture of the patient with more than one major handicap.

I have a suspicion, which I hope is wrong, that there are still people who, knowing the diagnoses, remain casual and unenthusiastic about treating the hearing loss in such patients. There are still, in fact, those who say 'What does it matter?' I can only hope that the few words at the end of this chapter encourage them to form realistic goals and then work for these with every means at their disposal. Enthusiasm, I believe, is infectious.

Chapter 17

OBJECTIVE HEARING TESTS

We have described the three usual methods of hearing test in some detail, as these are the tests which most readers use.

However, we have already said that some children who are either physically or mentally handicapped or severely emotionally disturbed, may not be able to cope with either distraction tests, cooperative tests involving speech, or conditioning tests, at the appropriate ages. It has therefore been necessary to find objective tests which could be carried out without needing the child's cooperation.

It has been known for a considerable time that sound produces electrical changes which may be monitored in several different ways. Initially it was shown that when an electroencephalogram was being carried out sound stimuli produced changes in the recordings, which could be picked out by those skilled in reading EEG patterns. However, this practice meant that the child had to lie quietly for a considerable period, the changes produced by the sound stimuli were small, and even the experts were not always very happy about their 'final' pronouncements. If sedatives or anaesthesia were given these might change the total picture of the EEG.

The next method that began to be commonly used, electrocochleography, was far more reliable, but its disadvantage was that the child had to be anaesthetized. In this method an electrode is placed through the tympanic membrane and rested against the promontory on the medial wall of the middle ear, produced by the first turn of the cochlea. This electrode could pick up electrical changes in the cochlea induced by sound stimuli. However, once again the changes were very small, and it was therefore necessary to use an averaging computer to summate the succession of small changes produced by the succession of sound stimuli. The result could then be recorded on an oscilloscope.

The third method devised was based on the principle that sound stimuli produced electrical changes in muscles all over the body. Obviously this derives from the alerting mechanism of the lower animals and the preparation for 'fight or flight'. It was found that a particularly marked electrical change could be picked up from the vestigial postauricular muscle behind the ear (see Chapter 4). This muscle which remains well developed in some animals who move their ears to locate sound is only minimally present in man. However, it is possible to put an electrode behind the ear, over this muscle, and use the electrical change produced by sound stimuli. As with electrocochleography each response is small, so once again, the responses have to be summated in an averaging computer. When this is done the total response to a number of sound stimuli can be demonstrated on an oscilloscope. In this case the sound stimuli used are clicks, with a wide-band frequency, having a peak at 4 kHz; 128 clicks are used, in bursts at gradually decreasing volume.

When a sound is perceived the nerve stimulus proceeds, via the 8th nerve, to the cochlear nucleus (see Chapter 4). From here some of the stimuli proceed direct to the 7th nerve nucleus on the same side of the brain. But it was found that, when sound was fed into one ear only, electrical changes could be picked up from the posterior auricular muscles on *both* sides. Obviously, therefore, some stimuli pass across to the 7th nerve nucleus on the opposite side of the brain.

Hence this form of test became known as the *Crossed Acoustic Response Test* (Figure 46)[1]. If any lesion interrupted the crossing pathway then the changes could *not* be picked up from both sides. In this way it was felt that this test could play a part in the diagnosis of neurological lesions, such as multiple sclerosis. It has now been superseded to some extent by the use of the various scanning techniques.

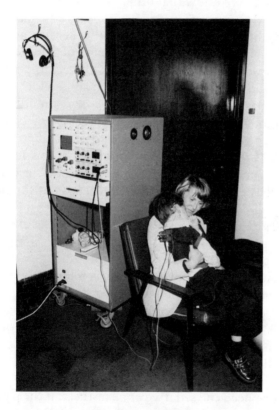

Figure 46   The crossed acoustic response test. Ellis Douek, whose research was largely responsible for this test, likes to think of it as 'an extra rattle' because of its speed and simplicity (see text)

The use of this test is, of course, very attractive because it is painless, quick, and does not require an anaesthetic. The writer at the moment is engaged on a long-term project to see how the results of this test done at a very early age, 6 weeks, correlate with clinical tests done at 7 months, 18 months and, finally, an audiogram at around the age of $3\frac{1}{2}$ years. This may help us to see, within limits, the usefulness of an objective hearing test done at a very early stage in an infant's life. We know that other factors affect the results of the crossed acoustic test. Results appear to be inaccurate in floppy babies, where muscle tone in general is not normal. They are also altered by the presence of 'glue ear', often disproportionately, and sometimes altered in severely retarded children, giving results which are too low. Although this test has been described in the very simplest way the number of synapses actually involved is, of course, not known, and it may be that the lesions causing the retardation also affect the synapses involved in this test.

In the meantime, the crossed acoustic test may be regarded as a useful adjunct to clinical tests. It should never be used alone, except in the very few cases where clinical tests are obviously impossible. In *all* other cases clinical tests should be made first followed by this simple quick procedure.

The latest electrical test that is becoming more popular at the time of writing is the *Brain-Stem Evoked Response Test*, largely because of the increased amount of information that it yields. In fact it has several advantages but its major disadvantage to those clinicians who see many mentally or physically handicapped patients is the length of time that is needed to carry it out.

The test needs no sedative or anaesthetic if the patient can lie still for a considerable length of time. However, as we have already said, the patients are often multiply handicapped and therefore not able to do this. In these cases either sedative or light anaesthesia may be used; a further advantage of this test is that the results are not in any way affected by these. Another advantage is that the test is non-invasive, although if anaesthesia is needed some otologists take the opportunity to double-check results by doing an electrocochleogram at the same time.

The positive electrode in this test is placed on the vertex of the scalp. Again clicks are used as the sound stimuli and usually 1000 to 2000 stimuli are necessary to elicit a clearly defined brain-stem response[2]. The same technique is used, with an averaging computer, as described in previous tests. The final wave-form produced is stable in shape, and it has been possible to prove that various components of the wave are produced at various locations on the auditory pathway. Thus wave I is associated with the cochlear nerve, wave II with the cochlear nucleus, wave III with the superior olivary area, wave IV with the ventral nucleus of the lateral lemniscus, and wave V with the inferior colliculus. There is still some discussion, however, about the significance of wave IV, and it is sometimes fused with wave V. The locations of both waves VI and VII also remain under discussion, although wave VI may be associated with the medial geniculate body (see Chapter 4).

It can be seen from this brief description that this test yields a great deal more information than previous tests described and this, no doubt, accounts for the enthusiasm with which it has been greeted by many otologists. It is also an extremely sensitive test for small high-frequency hearing losses, even those which have been asymptomatic in adults. However, when one considers the very large number of multiple-handicap children who really require an objective test of hearing, then the time, personnel and equipment required in order to carry out this test still seems daunting.

A chapter on objective tests would not be complete without mention of the *stapedius reflex*. It has already been mentioned that the function of the tiny stapedius muscle in the middle ear is to protect the listener from excessively loud noise, by cutting down the movement of the ossicles. It contracts when noises reach a level of around 70 dB above the listener's normal hearing threshold, so results showing stapedial contraction at around 85 to 90 dB are normal.

The measurement of the stapedial reflex is made using the impedance bridge, and results cannot be obtained in cases of chronic secretory otitis media (glue ear) where the middle ear is filled with thick catarrhal material, and middle ear movements are impeded by this.

We have already said that the use of the impedance bridge is to show the amount of movement occurring in the structures of the middle ear, at normal air pressure, at a negative pressure and at an increased positive pressure. If sounds of 80 dB onwards, up to 120 dB, are played into the ear the impedance machine should indicate the action of the stapedius muscle by suddenly indicating a decrease in the movement of the middle ear; for example, if the listener's hearing threshold is 15 dB at 500 Hz then the action of the stapedius muscle should be indicated on the machine at around 85 dB, whereas if the hearing threshold is 30 dB then the result cannot be seen until a sound of 100 dB is played into the ear. If the listener has a severe hearing loss then playing a sound of 120 dB into his ear does not cause a stapedial reflex as the necessary level above his hearing threshold has not been reached; for instance, if he has a 70 dB loss then only 50 dB above his threshold has been reached, which is insufficient to provoke contraction of the stapedius muscle. Therefore, in patients with a significant hearing loss a stapedial reflex is *not* expected.

On the older, manually operated type of impedance bridges stapedial reflexes can usually be measured at 500 Hz, 1 kHz and 3 kHz. On the newer automatic tympanometers, where the probe is inserted into the child's ear, a button is pushed, and a recorded graph is produced, the stapedial reflex at 1 kHz only is recorded. Such machines, however, are immensely useful, as the head-phones with the probe on one side and the pure tone played into the other side are only in position for a very few minutes, and can therefore be tolerated both by very young infants and also by very awkward, apprehensive toddlers.

Before we leave the subject of the stapedial reflex it must be stated that, occasionally, it *is* found in subjects who are known to have a severe hearing loss. This is due to the phenomenon known as *recruitment* which occurs sometimes when the cochlea is damaged. In this condition the difference between the hearing threshold and the level at which sound becomes painful is very much reduced. In normal subjects sound becomes painful at somewhere around 100 to 120 dB and, as we have seen, the stapedial reflex is evoked before this stage is reached as a partial protective measure. Thus in normal subjects there is a gap of 80 to 100 dB between the hearing and the pain thresholds. But when the cochlea is damaged this gap between hearing and pain thresholds may become greatly reduced, perhaps to somewhere around 40 dB, but the actual figure is different for every individual. But if, for example, the difference is only 40 dB, then a person with a hearing loss of 70 dB experiences painful sound at 110 dB, and the stapedial reflex can be seen at around that level. In some subjects with hearing loss the gap between the hearing and the pain thresholds is very narrow indeed, and this can lead to tremendous difficulties in the prescription of amplification. The commonest example of this, of course, is in the elderly patient suffering from the degenerative changes of old age, or presbyacusis. One moment he says that he cannot hear the speaker, but when the latter obliges by raising his voice, then the elderly patient says indignantly, 'Don't shout – I'm not deaf!' This commonly heard remark is not, as often thought, only due to the irritability of some elderly people but may be a sign of a very real and troublesome symptom. In the young child, one type of aid may give insufficient amplification, but the next type tried, giving only slightly more amplification, may produce complaints of pain on use.

If a child receives insufficient amplification from the time of diagnosis, and this state persists for some time, then the sudden use of correct amplification can also produce complaints from the young patient. His quiet world has suddenly approached nearer 'the norm' and becomes a very noisy place. What is more, he is now able to hear more speech and, consequently, more effort is required from him to produce speech. This is very hard work and, sadly, many children prefer to sink back into their quiet world with only their natural gestures as a means of communication. This is much less likely to happen if, after early diagnosis, correct amplification is prescribed, and the child is still *very young* when he is introduced both to speech and to the sounds of the world.

References

1. Douek, E., Gibson, W. and Humphries, K. (1973). The crossed acoustic response. *J. Laryngol. Otol.*, **87**, 8 (Aug)

2. Kavanagh, K.T. and Beardsley, J.V. (1979). Brain-stem auditory evoked response. *Ann. Otol., Supp. 58*, **88**, July–August, Part 2

Chapter 18

THE DEAF CHILD AND HIS FAMILY

From the moment of diagnosis, a deaf child's handicap is a family affair (see books by Bloom[1] and Courtman–Davies[2]*). In the initial stages the mother and father of the child need each other for 'the mutual society, help and comfort that the one ought to have of the other, both in prosperity and adversity' †. If this mutual help is not given by one to the other then only too often the marriage is broken by the dreadful blow of the child's handicap. Therefore at the moment of diagnosis adequate parent counselling should be available immediately, ideally from a specialized counselling service, but often from the visiting teacher of the deaf and the health visitor, possibly backed up by the doctor in the team at the centre where the diagnosis has been made. Unfortunately it also often comes too late, too badly or not at all, leaving two parents who are bewildered and stricken with grief and guilt. No wonder they reject the diagnosis and seek one opinion after another.

At the time of diagnosis the treatment of the parents is every bit as important as the treatment of the child. This is

---

* The author of the first book is herself the mother of a deaf daughter, while the author of the second is a highly skilled and experienced speech therapist who has helped very large numbers of deaf children and their families.

† 'Solemnization of Matrimony' from *The Book of Common Prayer*.

why it is vital that such children and their families are not seen as part of a busy, impersonal ENT clinic. A special clinic, with a highly specialized team, is essential if the parents are going to be helped to accept this very painful diagnosis. Rejection of it at this stage tends to persist, perhaps for many years, and means that the parents are unwilling to carry out the work with the child that is so essential at this stage (see Chapter 14). The child's future can therefore be severely and adversely affected.

The amount of help available to parents varies very considerably from one area to another. In some places the back-up help comes into play directly a diagnosis is passed on; in others specialized social workers play an invaluable role. There are considerable variations in the social worker service offered by different areas; one specialized social worker for the deaf, having special knowledge of the problems involved and special skills in the different forms of manual communication, etc., usually has to cover a very large geographical area and a very wide range of clients, including difficult adolescents, school-leavers and many elderly deaf people becoming more and more isolated and lonely. It is, therefore, often unreasonable to expect him or her to be able to spend a lot of time with newly diagnosed families. However, these families already know their health visitor and are forming a close relationship with their visiting teacher, so it is probably better from all points of view that the counselling should come from this team, in the absence of the 'ideal' parent counselling service. (This is probably yet another area where health visitor training could usefully be expanded. In fact it hardly seems fair that the potential health visitor should be expected to expand her knowledge in so many ways in such a short time. Perhaps there is a case for taking a long hard look at what we expect from our health visitors and how we prepare them for such a responsible and arduous job.)

When parents with older deaf children run into problems then the help of the specialized social worker should be sought without delay, as they can give invaluable help to multiple-handicap young people and their families. The young deaf adolescent also has very special problems. In hospital he no longer wishes to attend a clinic for 'children' but on the other hand he needs more time spent with him than the otologist can give in a normal, busy ENT outpatient department. I have, therefore, started special adolescent clinics, to try and bridge a difficult gap. The presence of a social worker at these clinics is invaluable in giving information about clubs, holidays, special courses and leisure activities. She can also give both practical and psychological help to those school-leavers who are finding it difficult to obtain or keep a job, and can create a link between them and the careers officer.

We have already summed up our goals but I would like to restate them for the last time.

(1) We want diagnosis before the first birthday in cases of congenital sensorineural hearing loss, so that treatment with amplification and auditory training can be established by the time the child is 1 year old.

(2) We want parents to be helped to accept the diagnosis by skilful counselling, and to realize that the treatment in the early vital years lies largely in their hands, guided by regular and easily available professional help.

(3) We want all hearing-impaired children to have the benefit of assessment by specially trained psychologists; who can give informed guidance to parents about suitable school placement for their children. (It remains astonishing to see how many hearing-impaired children are given psychological tests which are largely language-based.)

(4) We want parents to feel that they can discuss school placement with the psychologist, voicing their fears and apprehensions and being given enough time to talk these through.

(5) We want all children to have the best possible amplification, including radio-link apparatus of one sort or another where this seems optimal.

(6) We want as many children as possible to have the chance of using postaural aids, with open-minded teachers who are willing to experiment with the new modern types, being able to judge on results, regardless of any pre-conceived ideas or even possible 'built-in' prejudices.

(7) We want all children to develop as much speech and verbal comprehension as lies within their competence, and to have the *opportunity* of learning some kind of manual communication, should this prove necessary, either as an adjunct to their acquisition of good oral language (as it can fall into disuse as their oral language develops) or else as a main method of communication when oral methods seem to be failing. It is not intended, in the latter case, that oral methods should be abandoned, but the child should be provided with a method to make best use of his cognitive abilities, which is impossible without an adequate form of communication.

(8) We certainly want hearing-impaired children to have every possible and reasonable opportunity of mixing with their hearing peers – this, as we have said already, is good for all the children.

I believe that many hearing children would learn a signing system, given the opportunity. They would find it interesting, and the deaf children would be in the unusual and welcome position of acting as instructors and actually doing something better than their hearing peers. This would give deaf children a chance to excel, and most importantly, of course, every small advance in this direction helps to open up the closed world of the deaf. Surely this is the reason for all our efforts.

Reference

1. Bloom, Freddy (1978). *Our Deaf Children into the 80s.* (Old Woking: Unwin Bros., Gresham Books)

2. Courtman–Davies, Mary (1979). *Your Deaf Child's Speech and Language.* (London: Bodley Head)

APPENDIX 1: APPARATUS

Apparatus required for testing children is as follows. Obviously this can be modified by the amount of money available, but it is best to start with a little apparatus and add to it as money allows. It is *never advisable to substitute apparatus.*

(1) Apparatus for testing infants is found in the *Stycar hearing box*, available from NFER Publishing Company Ltd, Darville House, 2 Oxford Road East, Windsor, Berks SL4 1DF. This comes complete with the Manual for the Stycar hearing tests, an extremely useful little book, written by Dr Mary Sheridan. The *Nuffield rattle* is included with this set.

(2) The *Manchester rattle* is available from the Department of Audiology, Manchester University.

(3) A small selection of dolls' house furniture, with mother, father and child figures, a dog, cat, etc. is invaluable, and can be obtained from any good toy shop; as this is expensive, start with a small quantity and add to it bit by bit. Cups and saucers and teapots of varying sizes are also tremendously useful. (Larger plastic sets are useful for the 18-month-old child, while smaller china sets for toy table play are necessary for the older child.) A normal-sized plastic cup and a baby's hairbrush are needed both when testing for 'definition by use' and also for the *five-toy test*, as described in the text (page 75).

(4) The apparatus for the *Sheridan seven-toy test* (and also the *Sheridan six-toy test*), and the picture cards used in the *six* and *twelve high frequency picture tests* are all found in the Stycar hearing box.

(5) A boxed version of *McCormick's test*, suitable for children with a mental age of 2 years and above can be obtained from Barry McCormick, BSc, Dip. Audiol., at the Institution of Sound and Vibration Research, The University, Southampton SO9 5NH.

(6) Another alternative to the picture tests already mentioned is the set produced by Michael Reed and available from the RNID, 105 Gower Street, London, WC1E 6AH.

(7) The *free field audiometer* used by the author is manufactured by: Peters of Sheffield.

(8) The *sound level meter* used by the author is manufactured by Dawe Instrument Ltd., Concord Road, Western Avenue, London, W3 0SD.

APPENDIX 2: USEFUL ADDRESSES

(1) National Deaf Children's Society, 31 Gloucester Place, London, W1H 4EA. Telephone: 01 486 3251.

This society has active groups all over the United Kingdom, providing many useful services, mutual support, recreational activities for both children and parents and its own special 'Helper' scheme. These helpers call upon families and perform a large number of useful functions, helping harassed or depressed mothers in practical ways and providing emotional support in cases of need. It is strongly recommended that all families with a child who has a hearing handicap should join this Society. Local groups also make effective, necessary 'pressure groups'.

(2) Royal National Institute for the Deaf, 105 Gower Street London, WC1E 6AH. Telephone: 01 387 8033. There is an excellent library service available here.

(3) City Lit. Centre for the Deaf, Keeley House, Keeley Street (off Kingsway) Holborn, London WC2. Telephone: 01 242 9872/6. (For information on Paget-Gorman Signing Classes and also further education.)

(4) Kids National Centre for Cued Speech. Principal: Mrs June Dixon, 17 Sedlescombe Rd, London SW6 1RE. Telephone: 01 381 0335. (For all general and particular information on cued speech, particulars of tuition, etc.)

(5) National Association for Deaf/Blind and Rubella Handicapped, 164 Cromwell Lane, Coventry, CV4 8AP.

Telephone: Coventry (0203) 462579. New centre now opened at 86 Cleveland Road, Ealing, London W13, offering a particulary useful Mother/Baby Course. Full details available from this address. Parents are urged to seek this information.

Note: Freddy Bloom's book, mentioned above (page 224) has a large number of useful addresses, both in the United Kingdom and abroad.

INDEX

Index

Index

Index

normal impedence 192
and stapedial reflex 193
tympanoplasty 200
tympanotomy 185

understanding, development of 53
upper respiratory tract
infection 52, 183, 198, 199
Usher's syndrome 23, 106, 116,
117
Corti's organ in 119
incidence 24, 118
utricle 47

vasovagal attack 39
verbal comprehension 61
verbs, understanding of 164
vestibule disturbance 117
vocalization development and
deafness 157, 158
voice and distraction test 67, 71

volume of sound 29
measurement 34
vowels, low frequency of 30, 31

Waardenburg's syndrome 106, 204
components of 121, 122
Corti's organ in 122
hearing loss 122
heterochromia 121
intelligence 206
white forelock 121
wax
in deaf children 38, 39
and hearing aids 38, 39, 153
wax-producing gland 38
Wechsler Intelligence Scale for
Children (WISC) 33

X-linked gene 23, 105, 128, 129,
203
XYY syndrome 205